The information in this book is intended to help readers understand scientific issues and make informed decisions about their health. It is not intended as a substitute for treatment by or the advice of a professional health care provider. The authors and publisher have endeavoured to ensure that the information presented is accurate and up to date. However, they are not responsible for any adverse consequences that may arise from decisions made or actions taken by any persons who read this book. The views and opinions expressed by the authors in this book do not necessarily represent those of the publisher or of the organizations that the authors work for or are affiliated with.

THE FLU

PANDEMIC

AND

YOU

A CANADIAN GUIDE

—

VINCENT LAM, MD AND COLIN LEE, MD

DOUBLEDAY CANADA

Doubleday Canada and colophon are trademarks.

LIBRARY AND ARCHIVES CANADA CATALOGUING IN PUBLICATION

Lam, Vincent
    The flu pandemic and you : a Canadian guide / Vincent Lam,
Colin Lee.

Includes bibliographical references.

ISBN-13: 978-0-385-66277-2
ISBN-10: 0-385-66277-7

1. Influenza—Popular works.   2. Epidemics—Popular works.
3. Influenza—Prevention.   I. Lee, Colin (Colin Q.-T.)   II. Title.

RC150.L34 2006   614.5'18   C2006-902206-2

Printed and bound in Canada

Published in Canada by
Doubleday Canada, a division of
Random House of Canada Limited

Visit Random House of Canada Limited's website:
www.randomhouse.ca

TRANS   10 9 8 7 6 5 4 3 2 1

This book is dedicated to all those around the world
who work on the front lines of infectious disease.

CONTENTS

In the spring of 2003 I was launching a book. It was a novel called *Oryx and Crake*, set in a not-so-distant future in which a great many people have been killed by a swiftly spreading virus to which no one has immunity. Right at that time, the SARS outbreak took place, in—among other locations—Toronto, the city where I live.

My launch event in Toronto was cancelled, and elsewhere in the country people were alarmed when I coughed. Not only that, they were looking at me funny because of the epidemic described in my book. The events in *Oryx and Crake* were not duplicated in Toronto—thanks to long hours by Toronto health care workers—but nevertheless the fallout even from such a small outbreak of an unknown and highly contagious disease was frightening. Empty Toronto streets, empty hotels and restaurants, dead patients and health care workers, large financial losses—it was a hint of what might happen if something really huge got out of the cage.

If the human past is a key to the future, sooner or later something really huge will get out of the cage again. The Black Death changed history; the devastating flu of 1918–19 is recent enough to be a part of living memory. My own mother and the other six members of her family all caught it—possibly from my grandfather, who was a family doctor in rural Nova Scotia and treated many sufferers—though all survived. There are a lot of us on the planet, and we're in contact with other human beings much of the time. There are a great many other life forms, and each one of them harbours diseases. Viruses are like interplanetary travellers; life forms are their planets. At some moments the aliens invade, and we have no protection against them because we didn't see them coming.

The Flu Pandemic is about that moment—and about any pandemic moment. It's a calm, practical, and very thorough guide for surviving the alien invasion. Panic is our enemy, knowledge is our friend, preparation in advance is our best line of defence. This book even has food lists!

I know Dr. Vincent Lam and Dr. Colin Lee. I've travelled with both in the Arctic, where they were the doctors on Adventure Canada and Peregrine Adventures trips on which I was a resource person, so I've seen them in action during some fairly odd medical emergencies in remote locations. They don't fluster easily, and, young as they are—at least to my eyes—they've seen a lot of gruesomeness. Dr. Lam is not only an emergency doctor and a talented writer of fiction but a front-line SARS survivor. Dr. Lee's expertise in both public health and emergency medicine makes him uniquely suited for his role in pandemic influenza planning in Ontario.

They both know their stuff, and it's stuff you should know too. If you put it into practice, the life you save may be your own.

—Margaret Atwood, Toronto, 2006

CHAPTER 1

INTRODUCTION

In the spring of 2003, we were working as emergency physicians in a busy Toronto hospital during the SARS outbreak. Severe Acute Respiratory Syndrome was a new, life-threatening infection that appeared first in China in November 2002 and soon travelled to all continents except Antarctica. The world watched as the outbreak gained strength and momentum, infecting 8,442 persons in 32 countries and eventually causing 916 deaths.[1]

Within days of the first cases of SARS arriving in Toronto in February 2003, our vibrant, cosmopolitan city was turned upside down. Hospitals, the places people usually turn to when seeking relief from their ailments, suddenly became places that many people dearly wished to avoid. Some people who demonstrated signs and symptoms of SARS arrived in hospital desperate for help, only to discover that they probably had nothing more than a cold. In other cases, people who did have SARS but who were terrified of the events happening around them tried to avoid any kind of health care. Media reports alternately frightened and reassured people.

Toronto doctors, nurses, and other health care workers became ill along with members of the public, and some succumbed to SARS. Many health care workers in Toronto saw friends suddenly cancel all social plans, and in some cases, family members and loved ones became too frightened to be in the same room as them. Over 23,000 citizens of Toronto were quarantined as the infection spread. Restaurants were empty, Canadians were advised to avoid travel to affected parts of the world, and soon Toronto was placed under an international travel advisory, as each day seemed to bring a new round of infection, and a new chain of spread. Toronto, normally the third-busiest film production city in North America, saw shoots cancelled as actors and film workers refused to travel to our city. Hotels and restaurants were devastated by a lack of business, and people were sometimes seen going about the city in masks, causing those who were not wearing masks to wonder, "Are they overreacting?" or "Should I be buying some masks?"

Meanwhile, the doors of the hospitals had come to resemble the security checkpoints of a military facility. Access was controlled, and entry was limited to certain points for patients and others for staff members. At our hospital, the patient entry point was through a large, permanently parked Toronto Transit Commission bus that had been set up as a screening facility. Patients would go in one door, be assessed for their SARS risk, and then go out the other door of the bus into the hospital. At the staff entrance, there was a large and drafty tent through which we filed in a sombre line each morning, had our body temperatures checked, and received our daily supply of personal protective equipment.

A patient with a fever and a cough does not normally provoke a guarded suspicion, and certainly not fear, in doctors and nurses. During SARS, it did. Each such patient was someone who might have this potentially dangerous new illness, which had shown its capacity to transmit itself to the health care workers who came into contact with it. It was unsettling to be working alongside a physician colleague, and then to see her quietly excuse herself and ask for a temperature check, and a little while later to be evaluating her as a patient in an isolation room—with a fever and a cough. Fortunately, neither of us became ill, but our friends and colleagues did. A total of 109 Canadian health care workers were infected, and three succumbed to the illness. Most of them had the misfortune of being exposed early in the outbreak, before the full range of infection control procedures had been put in place. Thousands of people from all walks of life were quarantined and isolated, their family and personal lives turned upside down, in some cases their finances thrown into disarray by being unable to work. Then the outbreak ended. The onset of the last probable SARS case was in Taiwan on June 15, 2003.[2]

Now it almost seems like it was a bad dream. SARS was here, now it's gone. Scientists and the rest of the world wondered if SARS would be the next worldwide pandemic. It wasn't, and by the time SARS faded in July 2003, only three regions had taken the worst of this wave of infection: East Asia (China, Hong Kong, and Taiwan), Southeast Asia (Singapore), and North America (Canada). In Canada, we had 251 cases with 43 deaths. In that same year, outbreaks of the H5N1 avian influenza virus strengthened among birds in Asia, causing several cases of human illness. The prospect of an influenza pandemic entered the public consciousness slowly at first, but it has gained momentum in the media since then.

Many point to SARS as a success of the global public health system, because prompt and coordinated public health action contained the spread of a new infection. Other respected public health commentators feel that there were crucial infection control failures during SARS, without which it would not have caused the amount of damage that it did. Yet others propose that medical and public health systems around the world overreacted, causing a new set of unnecessary problems. There hasn't been a new case of SARS since 2004. On a worldwide scale the number of cases was small, and most people have never known someone who had SARS. Most of the people who contracted this infection recovered, and one could almost be convinced that we had somehow dreamed the whole thing. But the reason that a nightmare is frightening is that within its own confines, it is absolutely real.

Now influenza has taken over the infectious disease spotlight. Every day, newspapers run stories about dead chickens and the human victims of the H5N1 strain of influenza, which moves occasionally from birds to humans, where it can cause illness and sometimes death. It is feared that if this virus learns to spread easily from humans to humans, it may ignite a serious worldwide episode of human illness, a pandemic. The impact of SARS was tiny in comparison with the potential scope of illness and death of an influenza pandemic. Most experts feel that SARS was a useful dry run of our international and local public health systems— useful to show us how situations could be managed successfully, as well as how the outcomes could have been improved upon.

In a frightening dream, the most ridiculous and unexpected sequences of events flow naturally one into the other, and the conditions of reality twist into the logic of the dream. Familiar people, objects, and occurrences appear in dreams but somehow become exaggerated and inverted upon themselves to produce terror and dread. Working as a doctor during SARS was a bit like navigating such a dream. Fever, cough—these are the stock-in-trade of any doctor, the most familiar and simple of the medical problems we know. With SARS, a new, potentially fatal infection that had never before existed seemed to loom behind every fever and cough. At the start, no one knew what infectious agent caused it, or exactly what to do about it. Public health principles applied, of course, as did our knowledge of how to care for sick people . . . but what exactly was going on? The picture was murky.

As time went by, infection control and treatment practices changed with new information—the truth of yesterday was altered today. Toronto experienced two waves of infections. We lowered our guard after the first one, only to be hit by the second. This was a remarkable time to be a part of the emergency health system. Hospitals that, in normal circumstances, were occupied and utilized to their limit were suddenly forced to confront an entirely new biological threat. Hospitals were, in fact, a primary arena in which SARS infections were transmitted from one person to another. The challenges and responses to SARS crippled other non-SARS-related health care activities.

Working in front-line health care during the 2003 SARS outbreak did convince us of the importance of discussing these issues. SARS killed relatively few people, and on a world scale it ultimately had negligible impact when measured in human illness burden and fatality, especially in comparison with the potential impact of a worldwide influenza pandemic.

Nonetheless, it disabled health care systems around the world, resulted in massive travel disruptions, and interfered with thousands of people's personal liberties by way of quarantines and movement restrictions. Its impact upon societies was massive, although the scale of illness was actually relatively small. We were fighting in the dark, and we did the best we could. The next influenza pandemic may also cause its own dramatic societal disruptions. The potential scope of human illness that could be caused by an influenza pandemic is far greater than what occurred because of SARS, and the social impact is also correspondingly larger. As such, we feel it is important to discuss what we know about this issue in advance, and to make preparations for the next pandemic.

It is crucial to realize that we know much more about influenza than we did about SARS. SARS was an utterly new disease. Influenza pandemics have been occurring for centuries, and three of them occurred in the 20th century. Seasonal influenza is an ongoing and important health issue, and a close cousin of pandemic influenza. It would have been impossible to plan years in advance for SARS specifically, because no one knew it was coming. In contrast, the current concerns and awareness surrounding influenza and the attention paid to the H5N1 strain of influenza give us an opportunity to plan and prepare, drawing from the rich store of knowledge that exists about influenza.

There is no simple "right" set of things to do, but there are interlinked principles and issues that we believe are very important to consider. An infectious disease outbreak and the responses to it are a complex and nuanced affair, and in this book we explore both subjects with a broad view to large forces and principles, as well as a practical eye to the things that individual people can do in their own lives to address the risks posed by influenza. In a media climate whose spectrum of opinion seems to span everything from terrifying panic to a dismissive disdain of pandemic influenza concerns, this book is meant to give some sense of reality to what otherwise might seem to be the makings of a bad dream.

You could say that SARS, a new infection, crept up on us, but there is no reason for influenza to do the same. A nightmare terrifies because in its shadows lurk threats that are not seen. People and objects that are familiar have somehow become different—and so they hide dangers within them. In such dreams, we are afraid because nothing is what it seems. Then we wake up, and it is gone . . . which is how SARS is now remembered by many of us who were touched by it. Influenza is quite different, because it is always with us in its seasonal form, and its pandemic form visits humanity from time to time. Nonetheless, the shadows of fear always threaten to cast the familiar into the reality of nightmares—even if only in our own minds. In this book, we hope to pull pandemic influenza into the daylight, to lay it out for what it is, and hopefully in this way to make it less frightening.

Modern information technology and news media, which allow us to rapidly share information around the globe, are vital to a meaningful response to an influenza pandemic. Meanwhile, on a day-to-day basis, the remarkable volume of information regarding the threat of an influenza pandemic that is available in the world news media can almost overwhelm us. Yet, a single factually true news report upon this topic is usually not enough to give anyone a good understanding of the issues at hand. The facts that stream daily out of newspapers and the Internet really must be considered within a framework of concepts and a broad perspective upon the issues of influenza, if one is to appreciate them for what they are. This perspective allows facts to be meaningfully situated, often illustrates that there are as many questions as answers, and is essential in allowing us to ask the practical question, "What should we do?"

We believe that one of the best preparations societies can make for any type of danger, whether pandemic influenza or otherwise, is to have a knowledgeable and well-informed society and educated, wise decision-makers. This book assembles both current information and general concepts to help you understand the ongoing threat of pandemic influenza and the issues surrounding the H5N1 strain of influenza. It explores the ways in which individual and societal actions interact with infectious disease. It builds a conceptual framework for Canadians within which you can situate any individual news report, or a particular piece of public health advice, that may come in front of you. This book also contains practical suggestions on how you and your family can prepare for and deal with the threat of pandemic influenza.

CHAPTER 2

THE INFLUENZA PANDEMIC:
WHAT IT IS, WHY IT MATTERS

THIS CHAPTER IN ONE PAGE . . .

- History shows us that influenza pandemics are recurrent events, although their precise timing and severity is unpredictable.

- An influenza pandemic arises when a new strain of the influenza virus emerges that causes serious illness, is capable of spreading easily from one human to another, and has not previously circulated in humans.

- There is an evolution of risk leading towards an influenza pandemic. Modern scientific knowledge can allow us to better monitor, understand, and respond to this risk. This requires a timely and reliable global influenza monitoring system.

- At present, the H5N1 strain of influenza virus is worrying. It is becoming more widespread in birds, it has shown the ability to cause serious illness in humans, and the concern is that it may acquire the ability to spread easily among humans.

- In an influenza pandemic, all countries will be affected. Illness will occur on a greater scale than with seasonal influenza, and strain health care systems. Economic and social disruption is likely to be significant. All countries should make pandemic plans in order to reduce illness, death, and societal disruption.

- During an influenza pandemic, many deaths will occur but most people will survive.

PANDEMIC INFLUENZA: MANY FACES

What is pandemic influenza? Is it "just the flu," an illness from which most people are destined to recover? Is
it the dreaded "Spanish flu" of 1918–19, which resulted
in a global death toll probably greater than that of
World War I? Is it something that experts fuss about but
that might never materialize in your lifetime? Or is it a
threat to your personal health for which you should
make important preparations?

Pandemic influenza wears all of these faces. They
seem to contradict one another, and yet they are all
true. Each of these masks of pandemic influenza must
be viewed in terms of the forces and dynamics behind
its threat, and cannot be understood in isolation.

Pandemic influenza cannot be described accurately
in a newspaper headline. Individual news or TV items
either frighten us with headlines like "Sales of flu drug
soar amid pandemic worries" (CTV, August 2005) or
"Transportation system may screech to halt in event of
pandemic" (Canadian Press, March 2006) or make us
wonder if all the worry is misplaced ("Flu fears over
wild birds overstated," Reuters, November 2005).
Despite the factual accuracy of the majority of the popular media coverage of current influenza concerns, this
is a topic in which a limited set of facts can't suffice.
The concept of pandemic influenza is one that has

multiple vantage points, a natural and evolving history, a rich science, and implications for people's health. In reading one newspaper article or seeing one TV item, the crucial thing is to understand where it fits into the wider context.

Likewise, meaningful responses to this issue will not come out of fear and panicked reactions. Rather, they must be underpinned by a clear understanding of both what is known and what is unknown about pandemic influenza. Leaders and decision-makers must use strategically chosen actions to effectively address the risk that influenza poses in society. Individual people who seek to address the threat of pandemic influenza in their own lives must decide on a practical, day-to-day basis how to view the sources of risk to them, how these risks evolve, and how to take concrete steps to reduce these risks. All concerned need to appreciate what can be done and what can't be done about pandemic influenza, and must decide what is reasonable.

WHAT WE KNOW AND WHAT WE DON'T KNOW: AN OVERVIEW OF PANDEMIC INFLUENZA

An epidemic is a disease outbreak in which many people in a community or region become infected with the same disease. A pandemic is an epidemic that occurs over a wide area, such as several countries or continents. During influenza pandemics, an influenza virus causes an unusual and widespread amount of disease affecting many individuals, over many geographic regions.

When Will the Next Pandemic Come?

There will be another influenza pandemic. They are recurrent events. There is an evolution of risk in the events that lead up to them. The timing and severity of influenza pandemics are unpredictable.

What we know: Three influenza pandemics occurred in the 20th century, and they have a long history that reaches back into preceding centuries. The 1918–19 pandemic killed an estimated 40 million to 100 million people worldwide and decreased the average life expectancy by 15 years.[1] That especially serious pandemic was one of the deadliest disease events in human history. Subsequent pandemics were milder, with an estimated 2 million deaths in the 1957–58 Asian flu pandemic and 1 million deaths in the 1968–69 Hong Kong flu pandemic.[2] It is believed that a pandemic was averted in 1997 as a result of prompt animal control and public health action in Hong Kong. In 1976, a potential pandemic for which the United States made significant preparations never materialized.[2] The World Health Organization (WHO) now describes the evolution of risk leading toward a pandemic as occurring in six phases. As the characteristics and behaviour of a worrisome virus become more threatening the world moves from one phase to the next, with a corresponding increase in the risk of a pandemic. We currently have the scientific knowledge to begin to understand this evolution of risk, and to be able to recognize the events that signal a change in the virus's behaviour. The focus of attention rests currently upon the H5N1 strain of influenza, which is circulating in birds and is often referred to as "bird flu" or "avian flu."

What we don't know: We don't know when the next pandemic will occur. Changes in viral characteristics and behaviour may increase our risk in a stepwise fashion, but we have no way of predicting the pace of change. At the time of writing, we are in Phase 3 with respect to the threat of the H5N1 strain of influenza. If this strain does cause a worldwide pandemic, its behaviour may change so that we are suddenly faced with a virus of pandemic potential. Or it may take years for this or another strain to make the leap.

What Kind of Influenza Will Cause the Next Pandemic?

Pandemic influenza may come out of avian influenza, but they're not the same thing. H5N1 is one strain of avian influenza, and it presents the most important current threat.

What we know: "Avian influenza" refers to a group of influenza virus strains that circulate among birds on an ongoing basis and that can rarely infect humans. An influenza pandemic occurs when a new strain of influenza emerges that is capable of spreading easily from one human to another and has not recently or previously circulated in humans. People have little natural defence against such a strain of influenza. H5N1 is a strain of avian influenza that has recently spread from birds to humans in limited instances, causing illness. It might adapt into a strain that is easily transmitted between humans. This possibility is what gives H5N1 the potential to cause a pandemic. If this adaptation occurs, H5N1 will not be an avian virus—it will have become a pandemic-causing human influenza virus.

What we don't know: The H5N1 strain is an immediate and very important threat that must be addressed, but there is no guarantee that it will cause the next pandemic. The WHO, national governments, public health workers, and animal health workers on all continents are trying to do everything possible to prevent a pandemic. These preparations are important, whether it is ultimately caused by H5N1 or another strain of influenza. They will be applicable to whatever virus eventually causes the next pandemic, and H5N1 is clearly a worrisome current threat.

How Will It Begin?

The world may be on the brink of another pandemic. H5N1 has the ability to cause human illness, and if it learns how to spread easily between humans, this will be the start of the next pandemic.

What we know: The H5N1 strain of influenza has been closely monitored since 1997, when it caused 18 cases of human illness and 6 deaths in Hong Kong.[2] Since 2003, this virus has resulted in the largest and most serious worldwide outbreaks of influenza in poultry in recorded history. In December 2003, new cases of illness in people exposed to domestic birds with H5N1 were identified. At the time of this writing, over 200 human cases have been confirmed in ten countries, and over 50% of these people have died.[3] Most cases have occurred in previously healthy children and young adults. At present, the virus does not spread easily from birds to humans, and there is practically no spread between humans. If H5N1 evolves into a form that does spread easily from human to human in the way that "normal" influenza does, a pandemic will probably begin.

What we don't know: Exactly how any virus learns to spread directly and easily between humans is a subject of ongoing scientific inquiry. Individual genetic sequence changes within a virus occur randomly. The 'swapping' of genetic material between viruses may give a virus new abilities. These events happen at a molecular level. When a virus is widespread, as is the current case with H5N1, there is more chance for such genetic changes to occur. How and when they will occur cannot be predicted.

How Far Will It Get?

All countries will be affected. All should plan to implement strategies to reduce illness, death, and societal disruption.

What we know: Once a fully contagious pandemic virus comes into existence and a pandemic is under way, its global spread is believed to be inevitable. Border measures may delay arrival of the virus in a country but are not expected to stop it. Such a virus is expected to reach all continents in less than three months. People in all parts of society, in all countries around the world could be touched by this event.

What we don't know: Before a global pandemic, there are public health measures that may slow the evolution of this threat or possibly even avert a pandemic. Once a pandemic occurs, there are measures that should be useful for individual people, communities, and countries to slow the spread of the infection and to reduce illness, death, and societal disruption. Since influenza pandemics happen only every several decades, we haven't had a chance to try these things in the kind of organized way that will occur in the next pandemic, and therefore we haven't been able to fully evaluate how well they will work.

Who Will Get Sick?

Widespread illness will occur on a greater scale than with normal or seasonal influenza. We won't know many of the specific characteristics of the pandemic strain of influenza until it's here.

What we know: Infection, illness, and death rates are predicted to be higher than during seasonal epidemics of "normal" influenza. People will have little or no immunity to the pandemic strain of virus. A substantial percentage of the people in the world may require some medical care. No countries have enough staff or facilities to deliver medical services in their usual way when much greater than usual numbers of people suddenly fall ill, and strategies to care for sick people will have to change in response to the conditions of a pandemic.

What we don't know: Until it's here, we won't know the virulence—the tendency to cause serious illness and death—of the pandemic strain of influenza. We won't know its precise impact upon particular age groups. We assume that many of the pandemic influenza strain's characteristics, such as its incubation period (the time it takes for a person to show symptoms after catching it) and the period of maximum infectiousness will be similar to those of seasonal influenza, but we can't be sure until it has arrived.

Can We Slow It Down?

Medical supplies will be limited in relation to possible demands. This underlines the important role of public health actions in preventing and slowing the spread of illness during a pandemic.

What we know: As part of a public health strategy, antiviral drugs will have a role in controlling the spread of pandemic influenza as well as in treating individual people who become ill. The potential demands for these drugs may exceed the readily available supplies and stockpiles, so the use of these drugs may have to be rationed and organized to achieve specific goals. An effective vaccine for the pandemic strain of influenza has the potential to alter the course of a pandemic. It will probably not exist at the start of the pandemic and could well take several months to produce. All of this points to the importance of measures that can slow the progression of the pandemic and prevent or delay infection in individual people. Any delay of the pandemic's progression buys more time in which to produce medications and an effective vaccine and deliver them to people who need them.

What we don't know: We don't know how much benefit antiviral drugs will have in treating people who become ill with the pandemic strain of influenza, or in what groups of people or types of illness it will be most useful. It may be that antiviral drugs will deliver more benefit in preventing influenza than in treating it. The true assessment of the usefulness of antiviral drugs in an influenza pandemic can occur only once the pandemic begins. We don't know if and how quickly the new strain of influenza will develop resistance to our antiviral drugs. We can't be sure how long it will take to develop an effective vaccine against the infection.

How Many Will Die?

Many deaths will occur. No one knows how many. But most people will survive.

What we know: The number of deaths has varied greatly in each pandemic of the 20th century, ranging from estimates of 1 million in 1968–69 to as high as 100 million in 1918–19.[1] Death rates are influenced by four main factors: the number of people infected, the severity of illness caused by the virus, the underlying vulnerability of groups of people, and the effectiveness of preventive and curative measures such as medicines and vaccines. The pandemic of 1918–19 was more destructive than most, with estimates of between 40 million and 100 million deaths in a world population of about 1.8 billion. Clearly, this was a human tragedy of immense proportions, but even if we use the highest possible estimate of deaths in that time, 95% of people alive in the world at that time survived the influenza pandemic. Most pandemics are not likely to be as serious as that one, but even in the worst pandemic that we have on record, most people survived.

What we don't know: Accurate predictions of the number of deaths are impossible before the pandemic virus emerges and begins to spread. If a pandemic like the one in 1957–58 replayed itself today, the WHO estimates there would be between 2 million and 7.4 million deaths worldwide.[4] If the unusually destructive 1918–19 pandemic returned, some estimates forecast over 300 million deaths worldwide. Estimates of any such numbers are inherently speculative, and no one is able to predict precisely the events of the next pandemic.

How Will Society Be Affected?

Economic and social disruption is likely to be significant.

What we know: Because of high rates of illness and public health containment measures, people may not be able to go to work at various times. This absenteeism will affect businesses, institutions, and society as a whole. At certain stages of the pandemic, there may be international or regional travel measures and restrictions. These will contribute to social and economic disruption. A pandemic will run its course over one or two years, meaning that such impacts have the potential to be prolonged. It will be important for every country to maintain the provision of essential social services such as medical care and law enforcement, as well as clean water, electricity, food supplies, and supplies of essential goods like medications.

What we don't know: Social and economic disruption may be amplified because the pandemic may affect complex modern systems of trade. Modern economies are highly international and interdependent, relying upon economic partnerships and transport systems that span the globe. We expect that a global health crisis will require governments and companies to respond to worker illness and disruptions in supply chains, and possibly to take actions that may limit the movement of people and goods across borders or even restrict people from going to work at some points. It's hard to predict precisely how the world economy will be affected, but both economic production and the trade of goods may see changes. Although not all parts of the world may be hard hit simultaneously, the interdependence of economic systems means that disruptions in an industry in one part of the world may affect some linked industry in another country. Disruption may be most significant if events of a pandemic impair essential services, such as power, transportation, and communications.

How Should We Prepare?

As the risk of a pandemic evolves, a timely and reliable global pandemic influenza virus detection and alert system is vital for a meaningful response to these risks. The current efforts to monitor H5N1 build upon existing seasonal influenza surveillance systems. Meanwhile, countries, institutions, and individuals should plan their response to an influenza pandemic in advance of its occurrence.

What we know: The WHO works with national ministries of health and public health organizations to monitor circulating influenza strains—both those that circulate on an annual, seasonal basis and those that have the potential to cause pandemics. Since the last pandemic in 1968–69, the WHO's surveillance system on about 20 separate occasions has identified, investigated, and monitored influenza virus strains of pandemic potential.[5] A system that can rapidly detect changes in the behaviour of influenza strains is essential for a meaningful response, because different phases have a differing range of corresponding public health actions. Particularly in the phases that precede a full-blown pandemic, many of the public health actions must happen quickly and effectively in order to slow or potentially avert a pandemic.

What we can't know: We can't know when it will come, or how much preparation we will have managed to do when the pandemic starts.

SHOULD YOU BE SCARED?
THAT'S A PERSONAL DECISION

> *"To feel threatened by vague abstract forces—that's terrifying . . . When you've got an enemy, no matter how powerful he is, once he's been identified, you can get him in the sights of your guns."*
> —Donald Carveth, York University sociology professor, quoted in *Maclean's*, October 3, 2005

The discussion of potentially catastrophic events is unpleasant. Pandemic influenza is something that people find unsettling to consider, and this discomfort has at least two key elements. First, an event like pandemic influenza seems like a disaster that cannot be stopped or mitigated, like a tsunami or a massive earthquake. No one likes to think about unstoppable entities that have the potential to kill millions. Infectious disease is especially troubling to contemplate. It feels as if it springs up from an unseen and unidentifiable source and may come to us through our family, our friends, or simply a stranger whom we encounter. The second uncomfortable element is the prospect of seemingly random suffering and personal loss, through the illness or death either of loved ones or of oneself. Infectious diseases, especially new and menacing ones, carry the prospect of affecting people who are close to us.

We are mindful of several common perspectives within the discussion of any potentially catastrophic event that has not yet happened. Once such a spectre has entered the sphere of public discussion, some commentators feel that society should completely reorient itself toward preparing for the impending cataclysm.

They seize these ideas and predict something akin to the apocalypse. In online forums, some "flu bloggers" predict widespread chaos and complete social disintegration, as they trade tips on how to build Tamiflu stockpiles. In contrast, others contend that to forecast things like disastrous hurricanes, bioterrorist attacks, or infectious pandemics is inherently fear-mongering, overblown paranoia, or a waste of money, or perhaps is even a ploy to commandeer public resources toward some special interest group. Some things that we brace ourselves for don't happen—Y2K and its feared worldwide computing meltdown didn't really amount to much. These opposing perspectives are part of what has been described as our "culture of fear." In his book *The Politics of Fear,* the British sociologist Frank Furedi suggests that our culture incorporates a permanent level of anxiety, which turns its attention from one topic to the next—from global terrorism to earthquakes to hurricanes.

There is also a range of perspectives that follow any disruptive societal event. Often disasters look like human failures in retrospect. Following the September 11 attacks on the World Trade Center and the Pentagon in 2001, some declared that the disaster had been due to a failure of American intelligence operations, which should have detected and averted this threat. Following the 2004 Christmas tsunami in the Indian Ocean, people pointed at the lack of a warning system. After something terrible has happened, whether it is a tsunami, a bombing, or a pandemic, some people say in anger that experts either knew of the threat and didn't tell anyone, or didn't know but should have known, or that experts advised those in power—who did not sufficiently heed their warnings. Often a significant group of people feels, in retrospect, that some kind of negative event could have been prevented or that its effects should have been better prepared for and managed. Others resign themselves to human disasters as unavoidable tragedies, whether caused by terrorists, the forces of nature, or a divine power.

All these points of view, both before and after a disaster, usually contain an element of truth. Yet the choice of one particular perspective over another often seems to be a function of the commentator's inclinations more than the result of a well-rounded understanding of a particular issue. We make subconscious personal decisions in choosing a vantage point, having to do with whether we are inherently optimistic or pessimistic about the world and the potential dangers around us. Ultimately, we can each choose whether or not to be afraid.

The truth is that "experts" have some idea of bad things that may happen in the world but cannot predict the future exactly. We are doomed, therefore, to being either too worried about things or not worried enough. After a negative event, we can always say that there might have been better ways to handle the situation, and one's point of view may be related to whether one seeks to lay blame or would prefer to take a stoic perspective.

The Canadian Pandemic Influenza Plan, one of the earliest and most developed national pandemic plans, encompasses advance planning for a large and widespread international and national health emergency.[6] As all pandemic plans should, it acknowledges the unknown and focuses on practical actions to be taken. Before "something bad" occurs, what we must work with is a knowledge of the rough outlines of some kind of danger, often inherently lacking in specific detail. We believe the most important question is "What are the risks we can mitigate?" Instead of being excessively fearful or profoundly blasé about an issue like pandemic influenza, we think it's sensible to acknowledge that it does truly present a set of risks, focus our attention on understanding the implications of this phenomenon and its threat, and ask ourselves which responses to it are both practical and meaningful.

CHAPTER 3

SEASONAL, AVIAN, AND PANDEMIC INFLUENZA: THE KEY LINKS

THIS CHAPTER IN ONE PAGE . . .

- Influenza A and influenza B cause seasonal influenza epidemics each year. Through "genetic drift" and "genetic shift," the seasonal influenza strains change constantly.

- Influenza A also causes pandemics. All influenza A strains have their origins in birds, including pandemic strains that emerge every few decades.

- To cause a pandemic, an influenza virus needs to be new, or "novel," virulent, and contagious among humans. The current fear is that the H5N1 strain may be the next virus to fill this role.

- At present, H5N1 avian influenza outbreaks mainly in domestic birds are spreading worldwide but have caused relatively few human infections and deaths.

- Seasonal influenza causes deaths mainly in the elderly; in comparison, pandemic influenza tends to shift the burden of illness toward young adults.

- Avian, seasonal, and pandemic influenza are all inter-related in the life cycle of influenza and its interaction with humanity.

SEASONAL INFLUENZA

An epidemic is a disease outbreak in which many people in a region become infected with the same disease. Each winter in North America, we experience an "annual" or "seasonal" influenza epidemic. It begins in the fall, tapers off in spring, and is so routine that we call those months the "flu season." There is a spectrum of impact; a flu season can be mild, moderate, or severe. During this time, 5% to 20% of people become ill with influenza, with a peak of up to 30% to 50% in a severe season.[1] The flu shot, a key measure to address this epidemic, is an immunization that seeks to protect people against the most common strains of influenza that circulate in any particular annual influenza epidemic.

The effects of seasonal influenza upon people's health are well understood. Yearly, it causes approximately 3 million to 5 million cases of illness worldwide, including 250,000 to 500,000 deaths (mostly in the elderly).[2] In Canada, approximately 700 to 2,500 deaths per year are caused by influenza; it is estimated that 36,000 Americans die yearly from influenza and its related complications.[3] The Centers for Disease Control and Prevention estimates that about 200,000 Americans are hospitalized each year because of influenza, which extrapolates to about 20,000 Canadian hospitalizations a year.[4] In the United States, the direct cost for medical care of seasonal influenza is estimated at between $1 billion and $3 billion per year.[5] If one adds up the total number of illnesses and deaths caused by seasonal influenza during the interval years between influenza pandemics, these numbers are comparable to and possibly greater than the burden of illness of a pandemic.

Few people become upset because the flu season is coming, and most regard it as a relatively benign phenomenon. However, it does have important health implications, especially for those who are physically weak and vulnerable. In most people, having influenza means having a fever, a dry cough, aching muscles, and fatigue. It's not the same thing as a cold, which typically gives a person nasal congestion, sneezing, and perhaps a wet cough. A cold is a nuisance. In contrast, a case of annual seasonal influenza can leave a generally healthy person bedridden for several days.

Children become ill with influenza most frequently, but they rarely die of it. Infants are more likely than older children to develop serious illness. Healthy adults become ill with influenza, typically miss some work, and then recover. This is so common that we say that someone "just has the flu," which carries the implication that the person is ill but will soon be better. In a number of cases, mostly among people over the age of 65, people with pre-existing lung and heart problems, or people who are physically frail, it can have complications such as pneumonia and can sometimes lead to death. Frankly, society does not notice it as being unusual that frail elderly people with other health problems succumb to pneumonia. Although these influenza deaths are personal losses for families of the deceased, the phenomenon of this happening yearly as part of an annual seasonal epidemic is accepted by society as a normal event.

Influenza A

Broadly, two types of viruses exist, deoxyribonucleic acid (DNA) viruses and ribonucleic acid (RNA) viruses. They have somewhat different molecular machinery and building blocks. Examples of DNA viruses are smallpox and herpes; RNA viruses include influenza, SARS, Ebola, and measles. Of these two broad types, the RNA viruses have a greater tendency to change their genetic composition. Influenza is an RNA virus, and the types that affect humans are influenzas A, B, and C. Influenza B and influenza C are usually milder than the A type and are not seen to circulate in birds. Each year we see seasonal epidemics of types A and B in humans. However, only influenza A viruses have pandemic potential.

Most life forms have a mechanism to correct errors, or mutations, in their own reproduction, a proofreader that ensures that genetic material is more or less faithfully recorded as the life form reproduces. But RNA viruses, including influenza, lack such a mechanism, and their genetic material has a tendency to change as they reproduce.

Strains of influenza A viruses are classified according to proteins on the surface of the virus—the hemagglutinin or H proteins and the neuraminidase or N proteins. There are 16 H types and 9 N types. The genetic sequences of the RNA dictate the exact molecular structure of the surface proteins. This structure plays an important role in determining what species a particular strain of influenza A can infect and cause to have illness. For an animal or human, the extent to which its immune system can readily recognize these surface proteins determines how easily it can mount a defence against a particular strain of influenza. This recognition ability comes from an animal or human having been previously infected or recently immunized with an appropriate vaccine against a particular strain of influenza. Once it has had such exposure, an immune system has a memory that enables it to more easily produce antibodies against identical or similar strains of infection that it encounters. If a molecular structure is very new, or "novel," an immune system may have little or no ability to defend effectively against it. Some of the antiviral drugs that may be useful in treating influenza and preventing the spread of illness also act upon these surface proteins.

"Genetic drift," a process of mutation in individual parts of the genetic code, causes small and slow structural modifications to the protein shapes associated with an influenza virus. A person who is infected with seasonal influenza develops antibodies against that strain, giving his immune system more ability to defend itself by recognizing this strain. Genetic drift causes seasonal influenza strains to be a little different each year. These modified viruses may not be perfectly recognized by antibodies to earlier similar influenza strains, so the same person can be infected with modified strains of seasonal influenza year after year. If antibodies from a previous and recent exposure partially recognize a modified strain, he may have a milder episode of influenza.

Genetic drift is the reason why people who want to be immunized against seasonal influenza need to be vaccinated every year to achieve optimal protection. A global surveillance system monitors these changes in the human seasonal influenza virus strains. Each year, the three influenza A and B strains believed most likely to cause seasonal human illness are selected for the seasonal influenza vaccine. The annual influenza vaccine is about 70% to 90% effective in healthy adults under

65 years of age.[6] The effectiveness is somewhat less among the very young and the very old. Genetic drift is probably not the usual process that causes pandemics, but, as we shall see, some speculate that it may have a notable role to play in some circumstances.

In contrast, a process called "genetic shift" may suddenly produce a greatly different, novel strain of influenza. A genetic shift creating a new subtype of human influenza A is thought to result from the mixing of human influenza A and animal influenza A virus genes. In this process, whole pieces of genetic material may be swapped, conferring upon a virus the ability to cause illness in a new species. Such a genetic shift event may endow a virus strain that previously affected only birds or animals with the ability to also infect humans. That virus may be poorly recognized by human beings, who may have little or no immunity to it, such that it has the potential to cause a pandemic.

Conditions that favour genetic shift are those in which humans live, work, or play in close proximity to domestic poultry and pigs. Pigs are susceptible to infection with both avian and human viruses, and it was once believed that they were a necessary "mixing vessel," an intermediary for the scrambling and swapping of genetic material to create a pandemic strain of influenza. Recently, however, evidence is indicating that humans themselves can also serve as the "mixing vessel." This is one reason for the current level of concern surrounding the H5N1 avian influenza outbreak in both chickens and humans. If H5N1 can undergo genetic shift in humans without needing pigs as intermediaries, this increases the probability that H5N1 will acquire some genetic material from a human influenza strain that enables it to transmit easily from one human being to another, thus starting a pandemic.

Both "drift" and "shift" are constant, random processes of genetic change. Some of these events render a virus dysfunctional and no longer able to survive or reproduce itself. Others increase the ability of an influenza virus to reproduce and cause illness. When a virus is widespread, as is the present situation with the H5N1 strain of influenza, the frequency and variety of mutations are greater. This increases the chance of a dangerous genetic change occurring.

AVIAN INFLUENZA AND THE H5N1 STRAIN

Scientists believe that all influenza A, as a group of infections, evolved from avian influenza infections in the digestive tracts of wild birds. At some point, some strains learned how to infect other species and became dangerous in the lungs and bodies of other animals, such as pigs and horses, and eventually humans. It is hard to say when in history this jump first occurred, but human influenza pandemics have occurred for centuries.

At any given time, various strains of influenza A circulate among bird populations of the world and are called avian influenza. More than 100 identified subtypes primarily infect only birds. Most of the viruses are "low-pathogenic" and usually coexist with wild birds without causing illness in the birds or other animals. Sometimes a strain of avian influenza does cause marked illness in birds. When this happens, as is the current situation with the H5N1 strain of influenza, that strain is called a "highly pathogenic" influenza strain. In rare instances, an influenza strain may evolve to affect pigs, other animals, and human beings.

In 1996, after illness was observed in domestic birds in the southern Chinese province of Guangdong, a highly pathogenic avian strain of H5N1 influenza was found in a farmed goose. In 1997, there were outbreaks of this strain in poultry farms and markets in nearby Hong Kong. In the first known instance in which the H5N1 strain of influenza caused human illness, 18 people in Hong Kong became ill, and 6 died. All domestic poultry in Hong Kong was culled within several days, and there were no further human infections. In 2003 and 2004, the highly pathogenic H5N1 strain of influenza re-emerged to spread throughout Asia, causing illness in domestic birds in Korea, Vietnam, Japan, Thailand, Cambodia, Laos, Indonesia, Malaysia, and China. Japan, Korea, and Malaysia have been able to eradicate H5N1 from poultry within their borders. During 2005 and 2006, up to the time of this writing, there have been outbreaks of highly pathogenic H5N1 avian influenza in over 50 countries in Asia, Europe, and Africa, including rich countries such as France, Germany, Denmark, and the United Kingdom. It looks as if the disease will continue to spread, and some predict it will inevitably arrive in Canada, as early as the fall of 2006.

Domestic birds are much more vulnerable to the virus than wild birds. The first African outbreak, in Nigeria, saw the sudden deaths of 40,000 of 46,000 poultry at a farm. Over 150 million domestic birds have either died or been culled in an effort to control the outbreak of H5N1. This strain of H5N1 has also caused the illness and death of big cats like tigers and leopards, as well as over 200 cases of human illness. Three other avian influenza viruses have been documented to have recently caused illness in humans.[7]

Some experts speculate that the movements of the H5N1 strain of influenza follow the pathways of wild migratory birds, which would allow spread across long distances. However, it is unclear whether wild birds infect or are infected by domestic poultry. In many countries domestic poultry are raised in close contact with human beings. This type of interaction permits the occasional transmission of the infection to people. When more poultry are infected, more human cases of H5N1 also occur. It is theoretically possible for wild birds to transmit an infection directly to human beings; but this has not been seen, likely because of the limited contact between wild birds and people. One of the many strategies to control these outbreaks is to cull flocks of domestic birds. It is not recommended that wild birds be culled or interfered with, because of the likely ineffectiveness of culling and the detrimental effects on the ecology and environment of wild birds.

OTHER STRAINS OF AVIAN INFLUENZA THAT HAVE CAUSED HUMAN ILLNESS:

- **H7N7—2003, the Netherlands:** mild illness in 89 people and one death.
- **H9N2—1999, 2003, Hong Kong:** mild illness in two people (1999) and then one person (2003).
- **H7N3—2004, Canada:** mild eye infection in two people.

PANDEMIC INFLUENZA

Pandemics of various diseases have appeared over human history. A pandemic is a disease outbreak in which many people over a wide geographic area become infected with the same disease. Past pandemics include smallpox, cholera, and the bubonic plague, or Black

Death. Our most familiar and ongoing modern pandemic is HIV.

History suggests that pandemics caused by influenza A typically occur three to four times per century. There were three in the 20th century, the Spanish flu of 1918–19, the Asian flu of 1957–58, and the Hong Kong flu of 1968–69. Despite their geographic labels, influenza pandemics are not born out of geography. They arise from the constantly changing genetic character of the influenza family of viruses, and from the interaction between animals and human beings. It is thought that the genetic shift event that occurs between influenza strains found in birds and influenza strains found in human beings may give birth to influenza pandemics. A new viral strain that may cause a pandemic emerges when genetic changes give it three necessary qualities:

- **Novel**: A "novel" strain is one against which humans have little or no immunity or natural defence.
- **Virulent**: It infects humans, causing serious illness.
- **Contagious**: It spreads easily and sustainably among humans.

When such a virus becomes able to spread efficiently from person to person, it can travel rapidly around the world. It can cause higher than usual rates of illness and death, since people have little or no immunity to it.

A major reason that there is such a high current level of concern about the H5N1 strain of influenza is that it has met two of the three prerequisites to become a strain with pandemic potential. First, it is a novel influenza virus that has not circulated in humans. We have no immunity to it, nor do we have a vaccine. Second, it causes serious illness in humans, with an observed mortality rate of about 50% in people who contract it. The third prerequisite, the ability to easily spread from one human being to another, has not yet appeared. Human-to-human transmission of H5N1 has occurred rarely, usually involving very close contact with a sick person. To date, H5N1 has not spread beyond one generation of close contacts. H5N1 may be able to gain this last ominous characteristic through a genetic shift if H5N1 swaps material with a human seasonal influenza virus. This is the standard way in which it is believed that pandemics begin.

In a more unusual theory, some propose that H5N1 may have the potential to acquire the ability for human-to-human transmission through the direct changes of genetic drift. This process of adaptive change may happen in the course of H5N1 infecting humans. Although this is not the standard mechanism by which pandemics are believed to start, recent genetic sequencing of the H1N1 strain of virus, which caused the 1918–19 pandemic, suggests that this strain did not arise from a more typically expected genetic shift event. It may have resulted from a genetic drift event in a strain that infected humans and adapted to them in order to spread from person to person. Some experts fear that the H5N1 virus will take this postulated path of the 1918–19 pandemic strain and cause a severe pandemic.

Scientists wonder whether this adaptive genetic drift mechanism results in an especially virulent pandemic strain. This remains highly speculative research, in the realm of hypothesis requiring further evaluation. Not all scientists agree with this theory. It is one of the reasons that the current spread of H5N1 elicits serious concerns. The timeline of either a genetic shift or a

DIFFERENCES BETWEEN SEASONAL INFLUENZA AND PANDEMIC INFLUENZA

	SEASONAL	PANDEMIC
CAUSE	Influenza A, B, and C strains. C is the mildest.	"Novel" Influenza A strain.
WHEN IT HAPPENS	Yearly from October to April.	Three times in the 20th century; it's been 37 years since the last one.
WHO IS AFFECTED	Very young and very old people, and persons with chronic medical conditions and illnesses are at most risk of serious illness.	Everyone is at more risk of serious illness, and certain age groups may have higher risk: in the 1918–19 pandemic, young adults aged 20-40, and pregnant women were at a greater risk.
THE ILLNESS	Most people recover within a week or two.	Most people recover within a week or two, but there are more serious illnesses and deaths.
VACCINATION	Yearly vaccine is available and recommended for most people.	Vaccine is unlikely to be available in advance, but research is ongoing to make it available as quickly as possible.

genetic drift event happening in the currently circulating H5N1 strain is inherently unpredictable. It could take months, or years, or it may never happen.

HOW THEY ALL FIT TOGETHER

Pandemic influenza is a close cousin to annual seasonal influenza, but it acts differently. Historical experience shows that during a severe influenza pandemic, such as that of 1918–19, over 50% of people may be infected by the pandemic strain of virus.[1] During a typical influenza pandemic, most experts project an infection rate of between 15% and 35%. The virulence, or tendency to cause serious illness and death, of a pandemic strain is expected to be higher than for seasonal influenza. The pattern of illness may be very different from seasonal influenza, so that we see a greater burden of serious illness and death in young people when compared with the impact of seasonal influenza.

There is a fascinating relationship between avian influenza, pandemic influenza, and seasonal influenza. As strains of influenza A circulate in birds, they undergo genetic drift and genetic shift, and may acquire the ability to infect human beings. An influenza pandemic is caused by a strain of influenza virus that is genetically different from any that the human race has recently been exposed to. There is little or no immunity to this new type of influenza, and therefore more people become ill and die from it.

There are various theories regarding the unusual age distribution of illness and death during human influenza pandemics. One theory is that older people may once have been exposed to a strain of seasonal influenza similar to a pandemic strain, giving them some degree of protective immunity. Another theory is that younger people's immune systems may have an overly vigorous response once they recognize a completely unfamiliar strain of influenza, and this response may in itself worsen the illness. In either of these theories, the force behind the unusual age distribution of illness is felt to be the genetic changes in the influenza virus that underlie a pandemic.

Some scientists propose a life cycle of influenza's relationship with the human race, in which predominant seasonal influenza strains are periodically replaced via the phenomenon of influenza pandemics. It may work like this: A number of influenza strains cause seasonal epidemics in humans at some predictable level. Every few decades, a drastically new strain of influenza that previously circulated only in birds as an avian influenza acquires the ability to cause illness in humans and spread among them. This causes a pandemic, with an unusual amount of human illness throughout the world. In doing so, this new strain largely replaces the old strains that caused seasonal epidemics before the pandemic. After this, the pandemic-causing strain is something that most human beings have some immunity to, and it changes to become less lethal. Once this has occurred, the pandemic-causing strain and its future close relatives become the predominant circulating strains of seasonal influenza.[8,9,10] This continues for decades, until another new avian strain of influenza learns how to jump into the human species and restart the cycle.

In other words, avian influenza becomes pandemic influenza, which settles down into seasonal influenza, until another strain of influenza takes the stage. The behaviour of a particular viral strain may be as much a function of its relationship and history with animal and human species as it is a function of its molecular characteristics.

PUTTING IT IN PERSPECTIVE

Pandemic influenza has a different impact than seasonal influenza upon populations of human beings. That is a statistical observation that applies to large numbers of people. In one individual person, it may not behave differently at all but may even produce an identical illness. Seasonal influenza and pandemic influenza are actually close relatives in many ways and give most people fever, cough, muscle aches, and fatigue, followed by recovery. They are likely equally contagious. The difference is that in pandemic influenza, more people will have more serious symptoms, and a greater proportion of people may develop complications such as pneumonia and may die. For a single individual, it is impossible to predict whether this will be the case. An important historical observation is that although influenza pandemics are accompanied by an increased severity of illness and frequency of death in a population of people, it is also true that most people have an illness that is very similar to seasonal influenza, followed by recovery.

CHAPTER 4

WILL HISTORY REPEAT ITSELF? INFLUENZA PANDEMICS OVER THE CENTURIES

THIS CHAPTER IN ONE PAGE . . .

- Influenza pandemics have occurred repeatedly over the centuries.
- There were three pandemics in the 20th century. The first one was especially devastating, and the other two were much milder.
- In 1976, a pandemic was predicted, and a mass immunization campaign was undertaken in the United States to respond to this risk. The feared pandemic did not occur.
- SARS gave the world a recent taste of a global infectious disease outbreak. The rapid containment of SARS was an international public health success but does not guarantee a similar degree of success with an influenza pandemic.
- Some lessons from the influenza pandemics of the 20th century:
  1. Pandemics often give some warning before doing their worst damage.
  2. Pandemics tend to feature a "signature age shift," meaning that younger adults become seriously ill and die in greater proportion than in seasonal influenza epidemics.
  3. Pandemics tend to feature a rapid surge in the number of ill people.
  4. The pandemics of the 20th century have given us knowledge and insight to be able to respond more meaningfully to future pandemics.
  5. Honest and clear communication is the cornerstone of an effective response to a pandemic.

A Probable Influenza Epidemic, 212 B.C.

—Livys *History of Rome*: Book 25, The Fall of Syracuse

To add to their troubles both sides were visited by pestilence, a calamity almost heavy enough to turn them from all thoughts of war. It was the time of autumn and the locality was naturally unhealthy, more so, however, outside the city than within It, and the insupportable heat affected the constitutions of almost all who were in the two camps. In the beginning people fell ill and died through the effects of the season and the unhealthy locality; later, the nursing of the sick and contact with them spread the disease, so that either those who had caught it died neglected and abandoned, or else they carried off with them those who were waiting on them and nursing them, and who had thus become infected. Deaths and funerals were a daily spectacle; on all sides, day and night, were heard the wailings for the dead. At last familiarity with misery so brutalised men that not only would they not follow the dead with tears and the lamentations which custom demanded, but they actually refused to carry them out for burial, and the lifeless bodies were left lying about before the eyes of those who were awaiting a similar death. So what with fear and the foul and deadly miasma arising from the bodies, the dead proved fatal to the sick and the sick equally fatal to those in health. Men preferred to die by the sword; some, single-handed, attacked the enemies' outposts. The epidemic was much more prevalent in the Carthaginian camp than in that of the Romans, for their long investment of Syracuse had made them more accustomed to the climate and to the water. The Sicilians who were in the hostile ranks deserted as soon as they saw that the disease was spreading through the unhealthiness of the place, and went off to their own cities. The Carthaginians, who had nowhere to go to, perished to a man together with their generals, Hippocrates and Himilco. When the disease assumed such serious proportions Marcellus transferred his men to the city, and those who had been weakened by sickness were restored by shade and shelter. Still, many of the Roman soldiers, too, were carried off by that pestilence.

The 20th century experienced three pandemics, in 1918–19, 1957–58, and 1968–69. In 1976, there was enough concern that a pandemic might emerge from "swine influenza" that an extensive and well-coordinated mass immunization campaign was mounted in the United States, but no pandemic occurred. The influenza pandemics of the 20th century provide us with rich scientific data to understand the forces at work in each occurrence. Each of these episodes played out very differently in terms of the number of people affected and the degree of disruption in society. Since we have only these three pandemics to look at rigorously, and since pandemics embody a wide spectrum of effects, we are not able to make precise predictions about the severity of any future pandemic. Nonetheless, the pandemics of the 20th century contain important lessons, which we must understand in order to prepare for the future.

INFLUENZA PANDEMICS OVER THE CENTURIES
Early descriptions of what was probably influenza date as far back as Hippocrates, who recorded a likely influenza epidemic in 400 B.C. The historian Livy described what

was probably influenza in the Roman army in 212 B.C. Several episodes of widespread illness were described in the 16th century, though there is mixed opinion as to whether they were all influenza pandemics. Most medical historians believe that they were caused by influenza, given their rapid movement and the large numbers of people who became ill. The year 1580 brought what most agree was the first recognized influenza pandemic.[1] In the 18th century, there were at least two, and possibly up to six influenza pandemics of varying severities in Europe. There was a violent worldwide pandemic in 1781–82 that resembled the destructive power of the 1918–19 pandemic. The 19th century saw at least two, and some cite four influenza pandemics.[2]

1918–19: The Spanish Flu Pandemic

There are several hypotheses about the geographical origin of the 1918–19 pandemic.[3] One argument contends that it originated in rural Kansas. There was an unusual, severe outbreak of influenza in Haskell County, Kansas, in early 1918. A number of young army recruits from Haskell County may have brought this infection to Camp Funston, a crowded U.S. Army training camp, which was hard hit by an outbreak of influenza. From there, we can trace the spread of influenza to other U.S. Army camps, to other armies, through Europe over the course of World War I, and beyond. The H1N1 strain of influenza that caused this remarkable pandemic found its ideal breeding ground in crowded military training camps and progressed from there around the globe.

The influenza pandemic of 1918–19 had four waves. In the spring of 1918, an initial "mild" wave of disease was incapacitating but not particularly deadly, sending its victims to bed for several days. In the British naval fleet, 10,313 soldiers fell ill, temporarily crippling naval operations, but only four died. In April, Germany mounted its last major offensive of World War I, its last chance to win the war. At this crucial juncture, the German army faltered, with scores of soldiers weakened by illness, and General Erich Ludendorff blamed the failure on influenza. During an outbreak of influenza among the American forces in France, 613 soldiers were admitted to hospital but only one died. This wave affected most of Europe and reached as far as Bombay, Shanghai, New Zealand, and Australia. Despite its ability to prostrate young healthy men, this wave of infection killed relatively few people. There were so few deaths that British physicians writing in *The Lancet* wondered if the illness was actually influenza.[2]

The second wave began over the summer of 1918. Unusual cases of rapidly escalating and sometimes deadly influenza infections first appeared in healthy, young adults in the United States. In the fall, this more virulent form of the infection struck American army training camps, where thousands of soldiers fell ill and hundreds died daily, overwhelming the army's ability to dispose of corpses. This influenza brought fever, violent coughing, and sometimes bleeding from the mouth and ears. Some patients' lungs filled with blood and they died within one or two days. Others died more slowly from pneumonias and other complications, and many recovered. The deaths of army nurses and doctors created a widespread shortage of medical staff.[2] This wave swept most of the world. The worldwide case fatality rate—the percentage of people who died after becoming ill—is impossible to determine, but the numbers that do exist are unusually high, and frightening. In the American army camps, case fatality was 5% to 10%, depending upon the camp. In the British army in India, case fatality for white troops was 9.6%, and for Indian troops it was 21.9%. In previously isolated groups of people, the infection was more fatal. Entire villages in Africa, Asia, and Central America were wiped out.

Although no accurate data exist from many places, we know there were huge death tolls in large countries like India, China, and Russia. In Fiji, the flu killed 14% of the entire population in 16 days. In Labrador and Alaska, it killed an estimated one-third of the entire native population.[4]

The third wave in 1919 was milder by comparison, but it still caused deaths. In 1920, there was a fourth wave. Estimates of the worldwide number of deaths over the entire pandemic range from 40 million to 100 million.[4] The understanding that this event had been caused by a virus, or even the knowledge that viruses existed, was not achieved until years later. In fact, a bacterium that we now call *Hemophilus influenzae* bears this name because a German scientist, Richard Pfeiffer, had been firmly convinced, in error, that it was the cause of the pandemic and named it accordingly.[2]

1957–58: The Asian Flu Pandemic

The H2N2 strain of influenza, which caused the 1957–58 influenza pandemic, originated in Yunan province in southwest China.[4] It was recognized in April 1957, when it infected 250,000 people in Hong Kong. The peak number of worldwide deaths did not occur until October of 1957. It was over three waves that the

HISTORY OF INFLUENZA PANDEMICS AND OUTBREAKS

DATE	ORIGIN	DESCRIPTION	STRAIN
400 B.C.	Perinthus, Greece	Possibly influenza, but not a pandemic. Hippocrates records an outbreak of cough and pneumonia.	Not known
212 B.C.	Roman army	Possibly influenza, but not a pandemic. Historian Livy describes an infectious disease in the Roman army.[a]	Not known
855	Central Asia	Possibly influenza, but not a pandemic. Ebn-al-Atir describes a virulent epidemic that started in Central Asia in 855–56 and spread across Persia, killing many.[b]	Not known
1557	Europe	Possibly a pandemic.	Not known
1580	Asia	First pandemic. All of Europe infected within six months and then spread to North America. Illness rates were high—commonly agreed as the first influenza pandemic.[c]	Not known
1729–32	Russia	Pandemic. All of Europe infected within six months and travelled the known world with later waves more severe than the first.[c]	Not known
1781–82	China	Severe 1918-like pandemic. From China, it spread to Russia and encircled Europe in eight months. The attack rate was high, especially in young adults. At the peak of the pandemic, 30,000 fell ill each day in St. Petersburg, and two-thirds of the population of Rome became ill.[c]	Not known

1830–33	China	Mild to moderate pandemic. From China, it spread southward to the Philippines, India, and Indonesia, and across Russia into Europe.[c] Attack rate was high at 20% to 25% but mortality low.[c]	Not known
1889–90	Russia	Moderate pandemic. Called the "Russian Flu," from central Asia, it spread through Russia and Europe. The first wave was relatively mild, with low mortality, but the subsequent three waves were more severe. About 250,000 died in Europe, and the world death total was about two to three times that.[e]	H2N2
1918–20	Kansas, U.S.	Severe pandemic. The "Spanish flu" killed 40 to 100 million people, equivalent to 175 to 350 million given today's population. It killed more people than World War I.[f]	H1N1
1957–58	Yunan, South-west China	Moderate pandemic. The "Asian flu" killed about 2 million people, equivalent to 4 million given today's population. It spread across the globe in six months.[f]	H2N2
1968–69	Hong Kong	Moderate pandemic. The "Hong Kong flu" killed about 1 million people.[f]	H3N2
1976	Fort Dix, New Jersey, U.S.	False pandemic alarm, novel swine influenza: 230 soldiers infected, with 1 death; over 45 million vaccinated.	H1N1

a http://mcadams.posc.mu.edu/txt/ah/Livy/Livy25.html#Livy.hist.25.26

b http://www.iranica.com/articles/supp4/Influenza.html

c Potter, C.W. "A History of Influenza." *Journal of Applied Microbiology*, 2001; 91:572–79

d Patterson, K.D. (1987) *Pandemic Influenza 1700–1900: A Study in Historical Epidemiology*. New Jersey: Rowman & Littlefield.

e Dowdle, W.R. "Influenza A Virus Recycling Revisited." Bulletin of the World Health Organization. 1999; 77(10):820–8.

f Knobler, S.L., Mack A, Mahmoud A, Lemon SM, Editors. "The Threat of Pandemic Influenza: Are We Ready?: Workshop Summary / Prepared for the Forum on Microbial Threats, Board on Global Health." National Academy of Sciences, 2005.

1957–58 pandemic caused a higher than normal number of illnesses and fatalities. Around 2 million people died worldwide.[3] This pandemic was considered to be "moderate" in severity.

Advances in science since the previous pandemic allowed the 1957 pandemic virus to be quickly identified, and six U.S.-based pharmaceutical companies were convinced by the American researcher Maurice Hilleman to produce vaccine against this strain of virus for the American population. In the United States, the Asian flu caused small outbreaks in the summer of 1957. This was followed by widespread outbreaks in the fall, which were believed to have been accelerated by children returning to school, spreading the virus in classrooms, and bringing the infection home to their families. The first doses of vaccine became available in September, but by the time the pandemic had peaked in mid-October, fewer than half of the 60 million doses produced had been delivered. During this pandemic, 20 million Americans were infected and 70,000 died. The vaccine is believed to have prevented illness and death in many Americans, although it would have had an even greater effect if it had been distributed more widely before the peak of the pandemic.

Many planning exercises use the 1957–58 pandemic as the reference point for projections of the next pandemic. It may be a reasonable choice, since this pandemic was milder than the one of 1918–19 and more severe than that of 1968–69, but its middle status does not give projections from this pandemic any particular predictive value. It is simply a middle ground to use as a point of departure for planning.

1968–69: The Hong Kong Flu Pandemic

Hong Kong is thought to be the place of origin of the H3N2 strain of influenza, which caused the third 20th-century pandemic. After this strain of influenza emerged, it took about two months to reach Europe and the United States. In Europe, it did not cause an excessive number of deaths during the winter of 1968–69, and it was a full year later that mortality from this pandemic reached its peak. Interestingly, this pandemic behaved differently in the United States. There it caused a substantial increase in the number of illnesses and deaths due to influenza during the winter of 1968–69. This pandemic was unusually mild, with about 1 million deaths worldwide.[5]

Once again, a vaccine was produced in the United States, but it did not become available until one month after the outbreaks had peaked. This unusually mild pandemic was caused by a virus very similar to the 1957–58 virus, and so it may be that many people had partial immunity from having been exposed to the 1957–58 strain.

1976: The "Swine Flu"—A Pandemic That Never Came

In early 1976, a new H1N1 strain of influenza virus that was thought to have originated in pigs infected around 230 soldiers at Fort Dix, New Jersey. Called the "swine flu," it caused severe illness in 13 soldiers and one death.[6] There was rapid recognition and assessment of the outbreak and excellent collaboration among military doctors, public laboratories, and public health decision-makers.

The Advisory Committee on Immunization Practices of the United States Public Health Service assessed the scientific information that had been gathered and concluded that a pandemic was a possibility. Several important facts were considered: There was some evidence that this novel influenza strain had been transmitted from person to person, causing serious illness. People less than 50 years old had no antibodies, and therefore no natural immunity to this strain. Early detection meant there was enough time to potentially produce a vaccine to protect people. There was a good safety record for influenza vaccines, as well as for a military vaccine that had for years incorporated H1N1.[6] If we were to apply the current WHO classification scheme, which traces the evolution of a pandemic through six phases (and will be discussed in detail in a later chapter), swine flu would have been considered to be at Phase 5 at the time the decision was made to pursue this immunization campaign. Phase 6 constitutes a full-fledged pandemic.

Weighing this information, the American government decided to pursue widespread immunization of the American population, whom they judged to be at risk from this new infection. Once the vaccine was produced, 45 million people were vaccinated over the course of 10 weeks. Canada also participated in this immunization campaign, with some Canadians receiving this vaccine in November of 1976.

This vaccination campaign was both well implemented and monitored, and among those vaccinated, approximately 500 cases of Guillain-Barré syndrome were reported, although not confirmed. This is about one case in 90,000 people vaccinated.[7-8] This syndrome is a neurologic condition whose causes are not entirely clear, and which typically occurs in the general population at a rate of about one to three in 100,000 people independent of immunization. This is an incidence similar to that which was observed in those who received the H1N1 vaccination.[9] It has never been conclusively proven whether the vaccine did or did not actually cause an increased risk of Guillain-Barré syndrome. Nonetheless, the suggestion was made and it was a possibility. This, in conjunction with public criticism over the cost of the vaccination program and the absence of the anticipated swine flu pandemic, resulted in widespread vaccination being stopped in December 1976.[6] The vaccination of high-risk groups of people resumed on February 7, 1977.

If a pandemic had occurred, decisions regarding vaccination would have required balancing the possible risk of Guillain-Barré syndrome against the projected risks of the pandemic and the expected benefits of the vaccine. Since swine flu, the H1N1 strain of influenza, never caused a pandemic, it was easy to criticize the actions that had been taken. An article in the *New York Times* on December 20, 1976, dubbed it the "swine flu fiasco." Whether the correct decisions were taken in response to this outbreak of H1N1 is a subject that can continue to be debated. There is a strong case to be made that although the swine flu never became a pandemic, the decision to embark upon a large-scale immunization program was the right decision, given the available facts in the spring of 1976, and that it was the right decision because it erred on the side of trying to protect people from a potentially serious threat. Certainly it was not an unreasonable decision, although the anticipated pandemic did not appear.

WILL HISTORY REPEAT ITSELF? THE LESSONS FROM PAST PANDEMICS

Influenza pandemics recur. The exact way a pandemic unfolds has been highly variable throughout the 20th century. This variability is likely to repeat itself, with the next pandemic developing in unforeseen ways. In Canada, it will probably result in 4.5 million to 16 million people being infected with influenza. Between 16,000 and 1,120,000 Canadians will need hospitalization, with between 6,400 and 320,000 deaths. As you can see, this is a huge range, and it depends to a great extent upon whether the next pandemic is mild, moderate, or severe. A moderate scenario would probably mean 11,000 to 58,000 Canadian deaths.

Despite the significant differences during past pandemics in numbers of people deceased, extent of societal disruption, and characteristics of successive waves, there are common elements within the pandemics of the past century that can guide us in understanding the future.

Warning Signs

Past pandemics often gave warnings before doing their greatest damage, which occurred over successive waves of illness. We should heed such warnings in order to be better prepared for the next influenza pandemic, and we must understand the tendency of pandemics to act over several waves.

Some people imagine pandemic influenza as a cataclysm that will instantly appear, striking down millions of people overnight. Instead, history suggests that we will have warning. Since influenza pandemics play out in waves, with potentially greater damage occurring in the later waves, we may have some opportunity to prepare

ESTIMATES OF PANDEMIC IMPACT BASED ON A CANADIAN POPULATION OF 32 MILLION

	MILD SCENARIO	ESTIMATES FROM THE CANADIAN PANDEMIC PLAN (MODERATE SCENARIO)	SEVERE SCENARIO (1918-LIKE)
	Number (% of Population)	Number (% of Population)	Number (% of Population)
PERSONS INFECTED	4,800,000 to 11,200,000 (15% to 35%)	4,500,000 to 10,600,000 (14% to 33%)	4,800,000 to 16,000,000 (15% to 50%)
PERSONS REQUIRING OUTPATIENT CARE	960,000 to 3,200,000 (3% to 10%)	2,000,000 to 5,000,000 (6% to 15%)	5,000,000 to 8,000,000 (15% to 25%)
PERSONS HOSPITAL-IZED	16,000 to 32,000 (0.05% to 0.1%)	34,000 to 138,000 (0.1% to 0.4%)	320,000 to 1,120,000 (1% to 3.5%)
DEATHS	6,400 to 9,600 (0.02% to 0.03%)	11,000 to 58,000 (0.034% to 0.18%)	96,000 to 320,000 (0.3% to 1.0%)
ECONOMIC IMPACT	not estimated	$10 billion to $24 billion	not estimated

These scenarios are range estimates, based on the last three pandemics and the scientific literature we have encountered.

ESTIMATES OF PANDEMIC IMPACT BASED ON A U.S. POPULATION OF 285 MILLION

	MILD SCENARIO	ESTIMATES BASED ON GELLIN[a]
	Number (% of population)	Number (% of population)
PERSONS INFECTED	43,000,000 to 100,000,000 (15% to 35%)	43,000,000 to 100,000,000 (15 to 35%)
PERSONS REQUIRING OUTPATIENT CARE	18,000,000 to 42,000,000 (6% to 15%)	18,000,000 to 42,000,000 (6 to 15%)
PERSONS HOSPITALIZED	143,000 to 314,000 (0.05% to 0.1%)	314,000 to 733,000 (0.1% to 0.3%)
DEATHS	64,000 to 89,000 (0.02% to 0.03%)	89,000 to 207,000 (0.03% to 0.07%)
ECONOMIC IMPACT	not estimated	$71 billion to $166 billion

These scenarios are range estimates, based on the last three pandemics and the literature we have encountered.

a Gellin B. 2004. U.S. Government Pandemic Influenza Preparedness Plan. Presentation at the Institute of Medicine Workshop on Pandemic Influenza: Assessing Capabilities for Prevention and Response. Washington, DC: Institute of Medicine Forum on Microbial Threats.

MODERATE SCENARIO ESTIMATES FROM 2005 U.S. PANDEMIC PLAN	SEVERE SCENARIO ESTIMATES FROM 2005 U.S. PANDEMIC PLAN	SEVERE SCENARIO (1918-LIKE)[a]
Number (% of population)	Number (% of population)	Number (% of population)
90,000,000 (30%)	90,000,000 (30%)	43,000,000 to 142,000,000 (15% to 50%)
45,000,000 (15%)	45,000,000 (15%)	42,000,000 to 71,000,000 (15% to 25%)
865,000 (0.3%)	9,900,000 (3.5%)	2,850,000 to 9,975,000 (1% to 3.5%)
209,000 (0.07%)	1,903,000 (0.7%)	890,000 to 2,850,000 (0.3% to 1.0%)
not estimated	not estimated	not estimated

even once a pandemic begins. Each wave is anticipated to last about six to eight weeks. The spring 1918 wave of influenza caused a relatively small number of deaths, with the majority occurring in a subsequent wave six months later. The damage caused by the 1957–58 and 1968–69 pandemics occurred over the course of several waves in successive seasons. The pandemic influenza in Europe during the winter of 1968–69 was decidedly mild, but the wave of the winter of 1969–70 was more serious.[4]

We cannot predict the virulence of the next influenza pandemic's first wave, but if it follows the form of most of the pandemics of the 20th century, the first wave may be mild—a warning shot. The initial wave is not expected to be the only one, which means that from the start of a pandemic's first wave, we probably have several months to build supplies of antiviral medications, prepare vaccines, and undertake other important steps to prepare for subsequent waves. A vaccine may be available during the second wave.

These waves all constitute Phase 6 of a pandemic, the last in the WHO's progression of pandemic phases (which we will discuss more fully elsewhere). At the time of this writing, the world is in Phase 3, and we are strengthening our worldwide systems to detect when we enter Phases 4, 5, and 6. We are now better able to detect the progression of risk toward a full Phase 6 pandemic. Hopefully this will give us an opportunity for warning and preparation that was not available in the pandemics of the 20th century.

Age Distribution

Pandemics of the 20th century featured a "signature age shift." This means that there was a shift in the age distribution of deaths. Younger people had a sharply higher chance of dying from influenza than usual and made up an unusually large proportion of the deaths from influenza. We must consider the "age shift" in our current planning.

The typical pattern of seasonal influenza is that it kills the weak, the very young, and the very old. Pandemics behave differently. During the 1918–19 pandemic, the largest number of deaths occurred in people aged 25–29, the second largest in the group aged 30–34, and the third largest in the age group 20–24. In each of these groups, there were more fatalities than all deaths in people over the age of 60 combined. Pregnant women who became ill had a markedly high mortality rate, 23% to 71%.[4] During the pandemic of 1957–58, around 40% of influenza-related deaths were of people under the age of 65. In the 1968–69 pandemic, about 50% of those who died were under the age of 65.[4] Some of the possible reasons for these phenomena are discussed in the preceding chapter.

The impact of pandemic influenza on young adults is typically greater than the impact of seasonal influenza in that group of people. During an influenza pandemic, the risk of developing serious illness and dying might still be higher in an individual person who is elderly or has other health problems than in any individual young adult. It is simply that during a pandemic, a greater proportion of young people may fall seriously ill and die from influenza than would do so during seasonal influenza.

These observations have important implications for guiding the use of limited resources. For example, if there is a limited supply of medications or vaccinations, and priority is given to using those resources to minimize the number of potential life years lost, one may conclude that it is better to use resources for young adults and middle-aged people first, with the elderly coming later.

However, if priority is given to reducing the total number of deaths from influenza during a pandemic, the group of people most susceptible to serious illness and death would be the logical priority group for the treatment, whether young or old.

Young adults are in their prime working years. They constitute the workforce that produces and distributes food and goods, cares for children, the ill, and the elderly, maintains public services, and ensures public order. As a result, a disproportionate number of deaths in young adults has a magnified effect upon society. If an unusual number of police officers, health care workers, and employees in any industry are sick or have died, this affects others in society. Pandemic planning needs to take note of this, and all industries need to consider how they will function if an appreciable number of their workers are unavailable to work.

The Value of Delay

Pandemics tend to feature a rapid surge in the number of cases, with an exponential increase over a few weeks. During the 1918–19 pandemic, regions and individuals affected later during a wave did better than those affected earlier. From these observations, we can predict that delaying the progression of a pandemic may have great value, in terms of both the pandemic's behaviour and our modern-day preparations.

As the risk of a pandemic grows over the first five pandemic phases, we can try to avert it. Once we reach a full influenza pandemic, which the WHO would classify as Phase 6, it will not be possible to stop its worldwide spread. It is crucial to understand that once this happens, public health measures will be intended to slow the spread of a wave through countries and within a community but will likely not halt the pandemic. Nonetheless, slowing a wave of influenza may deliver great benefits.

Slowing a pandemic improves the ability of overloaded medical systems to respond. A hospital can better care for a thousand people with influenza over six months than it can help the same thousand people with influenza who all arrive on the same day. The manufacture of medications and medical care supplies is ongoing, and there is a finite number of medical care workers. It is easier to meet needs if there is a threefold increase in demands over several months than if there is a tenfold increase in demands over several weeks. In Canada we are fortunate to have a vaccine supplier, ID Biomedical (recently bought by GlaxoSmithKline), on contract that could produce up to 8 million doses of vaccine per month, once the vaccine is developed.[10] This means that during each day in which the progression of a pandemic wave is slowed, over a quarter-million more Canadians can potentially be protected by receiving vaccine.

During the 1918–19 pandemic, a city or area that was struck later within one of the waves tended to suffer less. In the fall of 1918, the lethal second wave affected the East Coast of America before the West Coast, and the West Coast cities had lower death rates. Similarly, people within a community, as well as soldiers in

American army camps, who became ill later as influenza passed through had fewer complications and deaths. Historical data do not suggest that this change was a result of improvements in medical treatment over time.[2] One of the hypotheses is that the H1N1 virus continued to mutate over the course of a wave of infection, and after a certain peak of destructiveness, the virus gradually mutated toward a less lethal, or less virulent, form.[4]

If, as historically observed, the virulence of a pandemic influenza strain decreases over time, slowing the spread of a wave may reduce the number of people who become seriously ill when they contract influenza. Even if this phenomenon does not repeat itself, delaying the progression of a pandemic will make it easier to meet the increase in need for medical care and buy us time to respond effectively.

Prevention and Treatment

The pandemic of 1918–19 occurred before scientists were ever able to isolate the influenza virus. There were no effective vaccinations, antibiotics, or antiviral medications. Today our knowledge and the tools that are available to address an influenza pandemic give us more scope for mitigating illness and death. Yet pandemic influenza remains an entity of inherently unpredictable risks.

Our understanding of pandemic risk is much greater than it was in the early 20th century. We recognize that diseases in animals pose risks to the health of humans. This gives us the possibility of modifying the interaction between humans and animals to avert or delay a pandemic. This will be further discussed in a later chapter.

When the next full pandemic arrives, we will have more fully articulated public health plans and tools than we had early in the 20th century for slowing its spread and mitigating its damage.

In 1918–19, many influenza victims probably died from a combination of viral and superimposed bacterial illness. Effective antibiotics and antiviral medications did not exist. We now have antiviral and antibiotic medications. During the 1957–58 influenza pandemic, only 25% of deaths involved pneumonia caused directly by the virus, while the remaining 75% involved other medical complications—typically bacterial pneumonia.[2] Although we cannot say with certainty what the effectiveness of antiviral medications will be in the next pandemic, we do have ample experience with the use of antibiotics for treating bacterial infections. Both of these tools should save lives in the next pandemic.

Effective vaccines did not exist during the 1918–19 pandemic. The impact of vaccines on a pandemic is potentially very significant, although it remains to be demonstrated in practice. In 1957 and 1968 vaccine manufacturers responded rapidly, but limited production capacity resulted in the arrival of inadequate quantities too late to have a fuller impact.[11] Currently, the world production capacity of influenza vaccines is small relative to the world's population and is centred in nine affluent countries, including Canada and the United States. During the next pandemic, we can predict that these affluent countries will protect their own citizens first, and poorer countries will unfortunately have limited and later access to vaccines. They may receive the vaccine only after the peak of the pandemic or not at all. This vaccine disadvantage, along with the already poor health status of those populations, may result in much greater numbers of deaths in those unfortunate countries.

The swine flu episode, however, serves as a cautionary and instructive story. That was in many respects a well-planned and implemented immunization campaign. The irony is that the pandemic never came. There is no doubt that influenza pandemics are a real and important issue for human health. However, they occur sporadically, and they don't necessarily act as we suspect they will, nor do they even appear when we think they are about to. During the 1976 swine flu episode, American health officials and their government acted in a timely, responsible, and coordinated way. They made decisions in the interests of public health that many observers still feel were the right decisions given the knowledge that existed at the time. The anticipated pandemic did not arrive. Although we now know a great deal more than we did at the start of this century, and we have much more scope to intervene in helping individual sick people and in taking broad actions for public heath, we still have to be prepared to accept that things may not go quite as expected.

Good Communication

One of the key lessons from the pandemics of the 20th century is that a lack of honest and public communication from government and health officials can seriously undermine a response.

The 1918–19 Spanish flu did not originate in Spain. That neutral country had an uncensored press during the war that reported on the first wave of influenza, which arrived there in May 1918. The term "Spanish flu" is simply a historical accident stemming from this being the first place that the pandemic was frankly reported by a free press.[2] Many other countries, in the midst of war, suppressed accounts of this worrisome disease out of worry that such news would harm fighting morale. This decision worsened the impact of the pandemic. Misleading and inconsistent government statements and media coverage undermined the public's confidence in government and were at odds with attempts to slow the spread of the pandemic. The director of public health in Los Angeles said, "If ordinary precautions are observed there is no cause for alarm." Two days later, he ordered the closing of all places of public gathering, including schools, churches, and theatres.

During that era, newspapers' objectives were often more about furthering their governments' political agendas, in what was viewed as a kind of patriotism, than about reporting the truth. In his comprehensive history of this pandemic, J. M. Barry writes, "Newspapers reported on the disease with the same mixture of truth and half-truth, truth and distortion, truth and lies with which they reported everything else. And no national [U.S.] official ever publicly acknowledged the danger of influenza . . . The government's very effort to preserve 'morale' fostered the fear."[2] In many parts of the world, panic was ignited as people saw their friends and family die suddenly and rapidly, while their governments urged them to not worry about any new illness. The pandemic of 1918–19 was destined to be a brutal and unusually destructive one regardless, but in many places poor public communication resulted in greater fear and social dysfunction. The damage caused by dishonesty and inconsistent public communication is recognized as such by public health practitioners, and is one of the crucial lessons that arise out of 1918–19. One of the core principles of the practice of public health is a commitment to clear and honest disclosure of health information to the public, and that is what we must expect for the events leading up to the next pandemic, and the next pandemic itself.

WE CONTAINED SARS. CAN WE NOT DO THE SAME FOR THE PANDEMIC?

In 2002–03 over a period of about eight months, a new infection now named SARS, Severe Acute Respiratory Syndrome, infected 8,442 persons in 32 countries and killed 916 persons.[12] It is widely believed that the outbreak was halted by aggressive and coordinated global containment measures that included the prompt isolation of cases and the quarantine of contacts. Does this make us confident of similar success in a future influenza pandemic with a similarly small cost in human lives? Unfortunately, it does not.

At first glance, SARS seems similar to influenza. They are both transmitted from one person to another via large droplets from our lungs. They are both respiratory infections that have the ability to travel across borders and oceans thanks to modern methods of transportation. However, there are substantial differences between influenza and SARS in their dynamics of spread. The incubation period, the time during which a person is infected with an infectious agent but not experiencing symptoms, of a typical influenza virus is one to three days. This is much shorter than the two to ten days seen in SARS. Influenza is most contagious early in the illness, typically between Day 1 and Day 3 of symptoms, whereas SARS is most contagious at about 10 days.[13] What makes influenza difficult to control is that it can be contagious about a day before the affected person even develops any symptoms.

What this means is that influenza contagiousness is at its peak just when someone is starting to feel ill. A person with influenza who has very mild symptoms may pay little attention initially, chalking them up to an "off day," while she has already begun to transmit influenza to others at work or at home and may actually be near the point of maximum contagiousness. In SARS, the point at which people are the most contagious is during the second week of illness. At this point, they are at their sickest, and are more likely to already be in hospital and isolated from infecting others. In addition, because the incubation period of influenza is much shorter, the virus is potentially able to jump from one person to another a little more quickly than the SARS agent.

What all of these differences mean is that in SARS, there is much more time for an ill person and for others to realize that they should be isolated than is the case with influenza. Influenza's characteristics enable it to spread more rapidly than SARS, without giving much time for people who are ill to realize that they are potentially spreading the infection, or for health officials to undertake the isolation and quarantine measures that were probably successful in controlling SARS. Addressing an influenza pandemic will be a greater challenge than containing SARS.

CHAPTER 5

PHASES OF A PANDEMIC: HOW A PANDEMIC COMES TO BE

THIS CHAPTER IN ONE PAGE . . .

- Public health is the branch of medicine that addresses disease in large groups of people. Public health pandemic planning and response seek to minimize illness, death, and societal disruption.
- A pandemic develops through several phases. The World Health Organization (WHO) defines six phases. At the time of writing, we are in Phase 3.

    Phases 1 and 2: interpandemic period

    Phases 3, 4, and 5: pandemic alert period

    Phase 6: pandemic period

- Public health actions seek to modify the interactions between animals and humans, between humans and their environment, and among human beings.
- Public health strategies respond to the changing issues in each pandemic phase.
- We may move quickly from one phase to the next although the pace is unpredictable. The earlier phases give the opportunity to plan and increase readiness for the next ones.
- In Phases 1 to 5, a goal is to slow the progress toward a pandemic and possibly avert a pandemic. In each successive phase, we are less likely to succeed in stopping a pandemic despite the escalation of public health measures.
- Phase 6 cannot be stopped and will run its course, with public health response aimed at minimizing illness, death, and societal disruption.

"The notion of trying to control a pandemic at its source would have been considered laughable just a few years ago— but that was before SARS transmission was controlled by public health measures. We have no idea whether a type A (H5N1) virus that was fully adapted to humans would continue to be highly lethal, but it is nevertheless incumbent on the global community to try to contain it."
—Dr. Arnold S. Monto, professor of epidemiology,
"The Threat of an Avian Influenza Pandemic,"
New England Journal of Medicine, January 27, 2005

PUBLIC HEALTH: THE POPULATION AS THE PATIENT

Most health care workers around the world are trained for and occupied with taking care of the ill patient in front of them. Treatments are administered patient by patient, symptom by symptom. An influenza pandemic causes individual people to be ill. However, its dynamics, movements, and growth affect large groups of people, so that the whole population becomes a kind of "sick patient." In an influenza pandemic each patient not only will be a sick person but will be a potential source of risk to those around him.

"Public health" is the practice of medicine that addresses the health of populations and the trends of illness in a large group of people. A public health practitioner monitors patterns of threats and illnesses and coordinates responses to them. The operating concept is that "the population is the patient," and the focus is on prevention. Pandemic influenza will be a rapidly developing problem with huge and serious implications for large groups of people, and a useful public health response will need to be correspondingly rapid and efficient. The tools of public health are not only pills or medications but also a mixture of social, environmental, economic, governmental, and health policies and interventions that aim to mitigate risk and protect large groups of people. Cities and whole countries may be the subjects of the public health responses to influenza. These public health measures may intrude upon people's lives in some ways, and it may be largely these measures that have a chance of reducing the number of people who become ill from influenza.

What Does Public Health Do?

In Canada, public health doctors work at the national, provincial, and local levels to address health issues in groups of people. The local public health unit, operating in a city or a small area, is in many ways the core of the Canadian public health system, although there is also larger-scale coordination.

Public health doctors address many of the same problems as clinical doctors, but they work from a different perspective. For example, a family doctor helping an obese child counsels her on diet and exercise. A public health doctor who sees a trend of increasing childhood obesity advocates for more physical activity in schools and nutritious lunches in school cafeterias. A doctor caring for a smoker helps him to quit. At the population level, public health practitioners have recently succeeded in implementing smoking bans in public places throughout North America.

Public health often addresses the interrelationships between:

- living environment and people: Mosquitoes can transmit malaria and West Nile virus.
- non-living environment and people: Smog causes lung illnesses, and extreme heat or cold causes deaths.

- people and people: People give one another colds, HIV, influenza, and other infectious diseases.

In human infectious disease including influenza, the concern is to prevent the spread of illness from the living environment, such as birds and mosquitoes, to people, and also from people to people.

PANDEMIC PHASES: AN EVOLUTION OF RISK AND RESPONSE

A pandemic requires efficient human-to-human transmission of a novel influenza strain to begin. This could arise from interactions between animals and human beings, and then between humans and humans. In the same way that a clinical physician is concerned about the interaction between an individual patient's heart and lungs, the public health practitioner is concerned about the interactions between animals and humans, and among humans.

The World Health Organization (WHO) defines three pandemic periods, which are subdivided into six phases. We are currently in Phase 3. This may all sound somewhat bureaucratic, but within this framework are core concepts necessary to understanding the pathway towards an influenza pandemic and the responses to it. The definition of each phase hinges upon the changing way that a new influenza virus strain spreads and causes illness among animals and people. Each phase is linked to recommended public health goals and responses that are targeted for that phase.

- **Interpandemic Period:** Phases 1 and 2
- **Pandemic Alert Period:** Phases 3, 4, and 5
- **Pandemic Period:** Phase 6

Interpandemic Period

Phase 1: No new influenza viruses have been found in humans.

In Phase 1, there may or may not be viruses in animals that are known to cause human infection. If such viruses exist, the risk of human infection is judged to be low. Countries should build the capacity for effective surveillance of and responses to new strains of influenza, in both animals and humans. The chickens and the farmyards need to be watched.

During all pandemic phases leading up to a pandemic, seasonal influenza remains an ongoing issue. Building strong systems to monitor and address seasonal influenza is important. In addition to addressing the important health implications of seasonal influenza, these systems often form the basis for surveillance networks and public health capabilities that are called upon to address pandemic influenza concerns.

Phase 2: No new influenza virus subtypes have been detected in humans, but a circulating animal influenza virus subtype poses a substantial risk of human disease.

In Phase 2, there are animal infections of viral subtypes known to cause human illness, but they have not yet affected humans. The distinction between Phase 1 and Phase 2 is based on what is known about the behaviour of particular virus subtypes. The goal is to detect and monitor influenza virus subtypes in animals that cause concern, to minimize the risk of influenza travelling from animals to humans, and to detect human cases.

The infection may need to be controlled in domestic animal populations by culling or immunizing flocks. Culling of wild animals is not feasible or recommended. There are a variety of methods of raising and working with animals that are understood to pose higher and lower risks of transmitting infections. The lower-risk methods should be implemented. Both the animals and the people close to them should be monitored for the presence of illness, so that if the virus jumps from animals to humans, the shift is quickly recognized. Both animals and humans in the farmyards need to be watched.

Pandemic Alert Period

Phase 3: We are now here, with respect to the risk from H5N1. There are human infections with a new subtype of influenza virus. Most of these infections are transmitted from animals to humans. Spread of the virus from human to human is rare. Each time the virus travels from an animal to a human, or from one human to another, this is an opportunity for it to adapt more to human beings and to potentially acquire the ability to spread from human to human.

At the time of this writing, the number of human cases of H5N1 is small, over 200 in ten countries. Most have occurred in Asia and Southeast Asia, and there have also been human infections in Iraq, Turkey, Djibouti, Egypt, and Azerbaijan. In most human cases to date, the infected person clearly was exposed to infected domestic birds, mainly sick or dead chickens.

In Phase 3, the virus is not easily transmitted from one person to another, and the instances of spread from one human to another are the exception rather than the rule. In certain rare cases the H5N1 strain of influenza has probably spread from one human to another via close contact.[1] In 2004, there were two family clusters of H5N1 cases in Vietnam in which human-to-human spread could not be ruled out, but they were considered to be explainable also by bird-to-human spread.[2] A family cluster in Thailand likely resulted from a critically ill girl who transmitted it to her mother and aunt while they cared for her in the home.[3] In the spring of 2006, an Indonesian woman infected with H5N1 may have transmitted it to some of the six family members with whom she was in close contact. Living in the same house or delivering health care to someone who is ill provides significantly more exposure and opportunity for infection than other interactions. These situations are the rare cases of human-to-human transmission of illness in Phase 3.

With every human infection, H5N1 has a new chance to acquire the ability to spread from human to human, potentially bringing us one crucial step closer to an influenza pandemic. Any single human infection is statistically unlikely to result in H5N1 developing this ability, but a greater number of individual human infections increases the probability that this may occur. The increasingly widespread outbreak of H5N1 in birds around the world increases the probability of these individual human infections, each of which is a kind of genetic Russian roulette. A crucial goal in Phase 3 is to curtail the opportunities for the virus to spread from animals to humans and from humans to other humans, and thereby to reduce the risk of a pandemic emerging. Those who are ill must receive high-quality medical care that takes necessary precautions to prevent the spread of infection from those who are ill to others.

As in Phase 2, farming practices that increase the risk that animals spread infection to humans must be curtailed. Preparations for a possible pandemic must be made in earnest at this phase, including scientific characterization of the virus subtype of concern, preparations for the use of antivirals, vaccine development, and building systems for public health response.

The Crucial Importance of Surveillance Systems

To know what to do, we must know what's happening. This requires systems to detect illness in humans, In addition to parallel systems in animals. Canada has a network of over 200 "sentinel physicians" who perform tests on people in their offices to detect seasonal and potential pandemic influenza strains, and to track influenza-like illnesses. We also need reliable laboratory systems. The Canadian National Microbiology Laboratory in Winnipeg can rapidly characterize influenza viruses as they are detected. Detecting the viral strains and clusters of cases that signal the progression to a different pandemic phase is absolutely imperative in order to guide public health actions.

Unfortunately, in most countries, surveillance and characterization capacity is poor, and there may be considerable delay between the appearance of a cluster of human H5N1 cases and the world learning of it. This is dangerous, because many of the possible interventions will probably have value only if implemented very early and very competently. Just as we in affluent countries need to have our own strong surveillance systems, it is equally in our interest to financially and scientifically support the surveillance systems of less wealthy countries. When a novel influenza subtype comes into existence that can be transmitted from human to human, the usefulness of any early public health interventions will depend a great deal on the early detection of this event.

In Phase 3, one of the essential containment measures is to isolate and treat individual people who become ill from the influenza virus of concern. This care typically occurs in hospitals, which is possible at this point because there are not many cases. Precautions and protective equipment should be used to protect both health care providers and patients. Regular handwashing is always a must. In Phase 3, contacts of people with a novel strain of influenza should be traced, monitored, and possibly quarantined and treated with prophylactic medications. Antiviral medications, such as oseltamivir (Tamiflu), are currently being used not only for infected patients but also for close contacts of patients with H5N1 to prevent further transmission. These measures are designed to contain the virus and to decrease the opportunity for the virus to transmit and adapt to humans.

Isolation and Quarantine

Isolation is the separation and restriction of movement of people *who are ill* with an infectious disease. **Quarantine** is the separation and restriction of movement of people *who are not ill* but who may have been exposed to infection, in order to prevent further transmission of disease. Quarantine can involve close contacts of an ill person such as family members, groups of persons who have been exposed such as passengers on an airplane, health care workers and other pandemic response workers, or even whole communities, using a widespread quarantine known as a cordon sanitaire.

Phase 4: There are small localized clusters of cases with limited human-to-human transmission. Although the virus has acquired more ability to move from human to human, it may not be very well adapted to human beings. The goal here is to contain the virus within an area, limit spread to possibly avert a pandemic, and gain time to prepare for the pandemic if the spread cannot be halted.

Phase 4 may be signalled by small clusters of human infections with the new virus subtype, without a clear animal source of exposure for all cases. Roughly speaking, there might be clusters of fewer than 25 cases lasting less than two weeks in a particular region, among whom some patients lacked contact with sick animals. This would suggest that the appearance of such cases is due to human-to-human transmission.

Phase 4 would see ongoing efforts to limit the spread of infection from animals to humans, as well as from humans to humans, and to contain the new virus subtype within the affected geographical area, delaying if not stopping its spread out of that area.

There should be globally coordinated attempts to delay or possibly avert a pandemic, while preparations are made nonetheless for an imminent pandemic. The world should do everything possible to aggressively provide early cases and contacts with antiviral treatment.

The Basic Reproduction Rate, R_0: A Defining Characteristic of a Virus's Behaviour

The cluster sizes of novel influenza cases that help us to decide that we have reached Phases 4 and 5 are estimates and not arbitrary. They come from statistical modelling of the expected behaviour for a virus with a given basic reproduction rate, its R_0, which is the number of subsequent cases generated by one ill, infected person in a fully susceptible population. The R_0 is affected by several factors including the infectiousness of the organism, the duration of infectivity of an ill person, and the number of susceptible people in a population that an ill person is expected to come in contact with.

The basic reproduction rate helps to predict the degree to which an infectious disease might spread through a population of people. For a disease to be able to spread, its R_0 must be greater than 1. If the R_0 of a novel infection is less than 1, meaning that each infected person infects on average less than one other susceptible person, this infection will fade from the population. If a novel virus has a low basic reproduction rate, although greater than 1, it generates smaller clusters of illness and has less potential to cause a pandemic. If a novel virus has a higher R_0, it generates larger clusters and has correspondingly more potential to start a pandemic. This is why the cluster sizes give us a strong clue regarding the imminence of a pandemic.

Many experts cite a R_0 of 1.5 to 3.0 for seasonal and pandemic influenza, in comparison with 8 to 11 for polio, 10 to 15 for measles, and 16 to 18 for pertussis or whooping cough. We can be thankful that the R_0 of influenza is not as great as those of these other infectious diseases.

In Phase 4, small clusters of cases are appearing, signalling that the character of the virus has made an important change in beginning its spread from human to human. In Phase 5, significantly larger clusters are observed, and the world is holding its breath before a full-blown pandemic starts.

Phase 5: There are larger clusters of human-to-human spread, but the cases are still localized in certain geographical areas. In Phase 5, the virus may be becoming better adapted to humans but may not yet be as easily transmissible as it could be. The goal is to contain and delay spread. This is the last real opportunity to avert a pandemic or to gain time to prepare for the start of a pandemic. Travel-related measures can be expected to be used to some degree, as will public health measures within communities to limit and slow the transmission of the virus.

Phase 5 may be signalled by larger clusters in the order of 25 to 50 cases lasting from two to four weeks. There is continued isolation of individuals who are sick, and quarantine of those who are contacts of sick people. Travel measures will probably be implemented by this time. In areas where there are clusters of cases community-based containment measures will be considered, which will be discussed in further detail later. We may see the establishment of dedicated influenza telephone hotlines and clinics.

Affected areas must offer care for the ill as well as limiting the spread of illness. Unaffected areas should strengthen their own pandemic preparations and if possible contribute to international requests for help. Individuals who are ill with the new influenza virus subtype will be isolated, probably in hospitals but possibly at home. The contacts of ill people may be traced and quarantined. Antiviral medications may be used to treat contacts in order to slow the spread of the virus and gain time to prepare in non-affected areas. Vaccine development efforts should be accelerated. International travel measures may be considered, such as giving health information to travellers, using health questionnaires for travellers, isolating ill travellers, and quarantining contacts. Travel measures may be used at international borders, but they may also be used within a country to try to limit or slow spread of the virus.

Phase 5 may involve a rise in the demands for health care as well as societal disruptions in affected areas. Economic systems and trade might be disrupted by travel measures. At this phase, it is appropriate for governments and individuals to have a high level of concern, and for decisive public health action to be taken. Meanwhile, panic and misinformation must be avoided.

WHO Rapid Response Plan

When the first clusters of "novel" influenza cases are detected, the world may have a chance to contain it. Mathematical models show that containment may be achieved through rapid and massive administration of antiviral medications throughout the outbreak area, in conjunction with area quarantines and other public health measures to contain the virus.

The WHO has a stockpile of 3 million courses of Tamiflu in Switzerland and the United States that can be rushed to the first affected areas to treat everyone in a geographic area. All of this hinges upon the outbreak being rapidly detected and confirmed, the government of that country quickly and openly communicating this information to the rest of the world, and immediately requesting the help of the WHO. The WHO's Global Outbreak Alert and Response Network draws upon experts around the world, whom the WHO aims to send as international field teams to the first outbreak areas of novel influenza cases within 24 to 48 hours of a request for help being made by a national government. Once the outbreaks begin, time is of the essence, and days count. Local governments will need to contribute key support, probably including the use of the local military and its expertise in logistics, transport, and the local language.

Modelling studies of this strategy in rural Thailand show that administering antiviral drugs to 90% of people in a 5 kilometre radius within two days after detecting illness in 20 persons should contain a novel influenza subtype with a basic reproduction number of 1.5.[4-5] The mathematical models show that if the containment strategy is to have any chance of success, drugs must be administered within 21 days following the detection of the first case. The most optimistic scenario would be that rapid and intensive use of area quarantine, other public health measures, and antiviral medications in the first outbreak during Phase 4 or Phase 5 prevent a pandemic. Such a plan has never been tried before, and its success remains to be proven.

Pandemic Period

Phase 6: There is increased and sustained transmission of a new and dangerous influenza virus subtype from one person to another in the general population. Up until now, the hope was to avert a pandemic, but this is no longer possible in Phase 6. Now the goal is simply stated but complicated to achieve: to minimize the impact of the pandemic. Isolation of sick people becomes a voluntary but still recommended measure. Individual quarantine becomes impractical and ineffective. There is increased use of containment measures for communities. There is more use of antiviral medications, and hopefully the quick and timely development, distribution, and administration of an effective vaccine. The specific measures that your government will take during Phase 6 will depend upon the severity of the pandemic as well as upon local issues.

Once we enter the pandemic period, it is virtually inevitable that all countries in the world will soon have pandemic influenza cases within their own borders. Phase 6 can be divided into Subphases 6a to 6e, which is a classification scheme we have adapted from the Australian pandemic plan.[6] In 6a, the "early" subphase, infections of the new strain of influenza are in the general population but only in certain localized areas of a country. In 6b, the "widespread" subphase, this influenza exists throughout a country and probably most of the world. In 6c, the "subsiding" subphase, the pandemic wave begins to subside. In 6d, the "subsided" subphase, there are no new pandemic influenza cases in a particular area for an extended period of time. Then, since pandemics typically come in waves, comes 6e, the "next wave" subphase, and the cycle repeats. The "next wave" will probably happen several months after the first wave.

At the "early" subphase, individual containment measures may still be valuable, particularly if a country still has only a small number of cases, perhaps imported. As the pandemic progresses, individually monitored contact tracing, isolation, and quarantine will be less relevant. Instead, people will simply be asked to stay at home if they are ill—a voluntary isolation measure. The numbers of ill people will be too large for the authorities to target measures individually; it would be like trying to stop an avalanche by grabbing the snowflakes with chopsticks. Instead, the focus will turn to community-based measures to delay and limit spread of illness. Large public indoor events such as concerts, hockey games, and shows might be cancelled. Schools and daycares might be closed. The most drastic though least likely action would be a cordon sanitaire, which would prevent entry or exit of any non-authorized person into or out of a community. International travel measures are not expected to prevent the spread of disease in Phase 6, but some such measures may be used to slow or limit spread.

Once Phase 6 starts, the race for vaccine development accelerates. Vaccine development occurs before Phase 6, but in Phase 6 this task has utmost urgency. Using our current vaccine technology, the final development of a specific pandemic influenza vaccine can occur only in Phase 6. A widely distributed, effective vaccine would alter the course of a pandemic. Once we are in Phase 6, all other measures are aimed at limiting the extent of illness, death, and societal disruption of the pandemic—in a sense, buying time until a vaccine arrives.

In Phase 6, governments will use antiviral medications like Tamiflu and Relenza strategically in order to treat ill people, give preventive treatment to the contacts of ill people, and contain disease clusters. Tamiflu and Relenza may be also used to prevent illness in essential service workers, such as health care providers and hydro, police, fire, and water system workers. There may be practical challenges in delivering health care in a rational, effective, and fair way; in preserving the distribution of essential commodities like food, medications, and fuel and essential utilities like water and power; and in preserving and maintaining trust and communication between public officials, health care systems, and the public. If there are law and order

PERIOD	PHASE	LEVEL OF INFLUENZA ACTIVITY
INTERPANDEMIC (months to years)	1	No new/novel influenza virus subtypes have been detected in humans. An influenza virus subtype that has caused human infection may be present in animals. If present in animals, the risk of human infection or disease is considered to be low.
	2	No new influenza virus subtypes have been detected in humans. However, a circulating animal influenza virus subtype poses a substantial risk of human disease.
PANDEMIC ALERT (weeks to years)	3	Human infection(s) with a new subtype but no human-to-human spread or, at most, rare instances of spread to a close contact.
	4	Small cluster(s) with limited human-to-human transmission but spread is highly localized, suggesting that the virus is not well adapted to humans
	5	Larger cluster(s) but human-to-human spread still localized, suggesting that the virus is becoming increasingly better adapted to humans but may not yet be fully transmissible (substantial pandemic risk).

GOALS AND RESPONSES

Goals: to strengthen global, national, and local pandemic influenza preparedness and minimize risk of transmission to humans.
Responses:
- improving farming practices
- enhanced animal surveillance
- early detection and Investigation of suspect cases
- consider culling and vaccination of animal sources

Goals: to rapidly characterize new virus subtype and contain virus.
Responses:
- consider culling and vaccination of animal source
- prompt reporting and isolation of human infections
- containment measures for individuals[a]
- use of antiviral medications for ill persons and consider use in close contacts

Goals: to contain virus within a limited area and delay spread.
Responses:
- continued containment measures for individuals, with increased use of activity and travel restriction, quarantine and antiviral medications for close contacts, and individual containment measures in order to gain time to implement preparedness measures in non-affected areas
- accelerate vaccine development efforts
- consider travel measures[b]

Goals: to contain and delay spread to avert pandemic and to gain time to implement pandemic measures.
Responses:
- continue containment measures for individuals
- continue use of antiviral medications for ill persons and consider use in close contacts
- consider travel measures
- consider containment measures for communities[c]

a Containment measures for individuals: a) For ill persons, isolation for five days for adults and seven days for young children (the anticipated periods of communicability or contagiousness) in hospital or home, and b) for close contacts, one or more of the following: tracing, monitoring, activity and travel restriction, and quarantine for three days (the anticipated incubation period of the virus, where the contact may be infected but not yet symptomatic) at home.

b Travel measures: possible measures include travel health alert notices, exit and/or entry screening, isolation of ill travellers and quarantine of their close contacts at border points, travel advisories, border closures.

c Containment measures for communities: possible measures include self-isolation, closure of schools and daycares, and restriction of large public indoor gatherings.

PERIOD	PHASE	LEVEL OF INFLUENZA ACTIVITY
PANDEMIC (weeks to years)	6a	Pandemic (early): increased and sustained transmission in general population but in localized areas in the country.
	6b	Pandemic (widespread): when containment measures for individuals and groups are thought to be no longer effective.
	6c	Pandemic (subsiding): after current wave peaks and pandemic starts to subside, with decreasing new cases, and possibly good vaccine coverage.
	6d	Pandemic (subsided) with no new cases reported.
	6e	Next pandemic wave or end of pandemic.

GOALS AND RESPONSES

Goal: to minimize impact of pandemic.
Responses:
- continue containment measures for individuals, but probably with the contacts self-monitored, instead of being quarantined, and where possible isolation of non-critically-ill individuals at home
- consider containment measures for communities as in 5
- antiviral drugs as per priority groups to treat those at highest risk of severe illness and death, and to prevent infection in those persons needed to preserve the delivery of health care and other essential services
- consider travel measures

Responses:
- containment measures for individuals as in 6a
- consider containment measures for communities as in 6a
- continue use of antiviral drugs as in 6a
- immunize when vaccine is available

Responses:
- consider discontinuation of community-wide containment measures
- containment measures for individuals as in 6b
- continue use of antiviral drugs as in 6b
- immunize when vaccine is available

Responses:
- active monitoring of high-risk populations for weeks
- immunize when vaccine is available

Responses:
- immunize when vaccine is available
- go to 6a or, if end of the pandemic, go to phase 1

issues, economic losses, and other societal difficulties, governments will need to try to mitigate them. These problems might not happen, but they're possible.

Some predict that the next pandemic will be a relatively mild event, with few deaths and little societal disruption. This may be the case, and this is the central goal of our pandemic response. Other commentators predict an apocalypse threatening the very fabric of society. This is unlikely; the worst pandemic of the 20th century, that of 1918–19, was catastrophic in its human toll but did not destroy the societies of its time. As the pandemic progresses through the subphases of Phase 6, the most effective ways to minimize illness and death may change. A pandemic is a fluid, evolving process, and the public health interventions require a corresponding alertness and responsiveness to the dynamics of the pandemic.

SOME PERSPECTIVE UPON THE PANDEMIC PHASES

There are several overarching concepts to keep in mind while considering the six pandemic phases and the relevant public health interventions.

Local differences: Each country must look at each phase with respect to its domestic situation and must consider where it stands within the global situation as it evolves.

These phases are international in concept and implication, but at some point some countries may have cases of the novel strain of influenza while others do not. Some countries may have clusters of cases at the same time that other countries are watching for the importation of cases. These differences require different public health actions, in accordance with local issues and priorities. We may see some actions occurring in some countries but not immediately in others. Because Canada is so big, there will probably be some differences in the occurrence of initial cases and, consequently, differing public health actions in different regions.

The public health dilemma: Earlier on, there is a greater possibility that certain public health actions will make a difference, but earlier there may be less political support for such actions.

Each country should focus considerable public health attention on the pandemic alert period (Phases 3, 4, and 5). At this point, it might be possible to delay or even avert a pandemic, and we have time to prepare. Once the pandemic period starts (Phase 6), the early days are the critical point at which interventions might have a chance of modifying the spread of a new influenza virus. Each country needs to be ready to act early, swiftly, and decisively with the appearance of new risks in the pandemic alert period and early in the pandemic period.

This concept is politically difficult, because in the pandemic alert period there are relatively few human infections and deaths, and there is an uncertain timeline of the progression through the pandemic phases. There is the difficult question of what amount of resources to devote to pandemic preparedness, when every health care system and country has other pressing issues to address. This is an issue that Canada and countries around the world are currently grappling with. There is great media attention, only a small number of human deaths, and a mounting risk of pandemic influenza. To some, it may seem like an abstract issue. It's not. It's a real issue, but the question for justifiable debate is "How worried should we be?" More pointedly, "How much should our preparations take away from other important investments in health and well-being that we make—as individuals, institutions, and nations?" No countries have unlimited funds. A sensible strategy may be for pandemic planning to overlap with planning for other emergencies, such as earthquakes, blackouts, or ice storms, since many of the basic principles of emergency preparation apply to all these events.

Public health interventions require extensive scientific, political, economic, and social cooperation. More disruptive interventions may be required in successive pandemic phases. The ultimate precise degree of success of these interventions is difficult to predict, partly because there are a large number of scientific variables involved and partly because they take place in the real world of political, social, and personal conditions. It's one thing to have the infectious disease and public health knowledge. Successfully translating that knowledge into useful individual and societal behaviour requires a high degree of convergence between science and people. It is fundamentally hinged upon the effective communication of sometimes difficult information.

Even once the pandemic period (Phase 6) starts, the numbers of people who are ill may be small at the outset, with the potential for large increases over time. This is politically problematic. Smaller numbers of ill people create less political will for socially and economically disruptive interventions such as isolation and quarantine or for other measures that may interfere with personal liberties. Later, large numbers of people falling ill and dying may motivate intervention regardless of societal costs, and possibly regardless of expected benefits. Ironically, once the pandemic is well established and the virus is widely circulating, certain actions such as mandatory isolation and quarantine, which would have had a chance of being helpful very early, will no longer be as useful. Certainly, they may no longer justify their costs even if widespread illness has allowed them to acquire popular and political support.

Inevitable progression: Influenza experts and the historical record tell us that each influenza pandemic phase typically evolves to the next, and then the cycle repeats.

Following the end of a pandemic there is a return to the interpandemic period (Phases 1 and 2), and it all starts over. Pandemic influenza recurs over centuries as a cycle of global human illness. Only in the past half-century has our scientific knowledge allowed us to even contemplate altering the course of a pandemic. We now know what measures may mitigate the damage of a pandemic or, in the most optimistically speculative view, prevent one. Since achieving the latter goal may be unlikely, much meaningful discussion should focus on damage control. Some do believe that the public health action of culling all the domestic chickens (1.5 million) in Hong Kong in 1997 prevented a pandemic. As each phase progresses to the next, some of the public health interventions in the prior phase will continue, some will be directly replaced by different interventions, while others will be rendered ineffective by the progression of the pandemic.

Uncertain timing: The progression from Phase 3 to Phase 6 could occur over years or within months, and it is inherently unpredictable.

We could endlessly prepare for each individual phase

and perhaps never be able to completely address the issues of each phase. The pace of progression from one phase to the next is dependent upon the molecular changes and infectious characteristics of the new influenza virus subtype, and they are unpredictable. Which countries are affected first will depend to some degree on luck. All eyes are on Asia for the emergence of the first pandemic cases, since H5N1 is well established there and that continent has many ducks, chickens, pigs, and humans living at close quarters. This creates the right conditions for the development of a pandemic, but there is no guarantee it will happen there. Once the pandemic starts, trade links, travel patterns, and random chance will determine where the pandemic spreads. If Phases 3, 4, and 5 are prolonged, this should be viewed as a great lucky gift and will provide our best opportunity to slow down or mitigate the potential damage of an influenza pandemic.

CHAPTER 6

CONTAINING THE VIRUS

THIS CHAPTER IN ONE PAGE . . .

- Travel measures are likely to be used in Phases 4 and 5 and possibly early in Phase 6. There isn't much evidence of these measures working in past pandemics, except in island nations. However, in past pandemics these measures were mostly attempted in Phase 6, and current thinking advocates their use primarily in Phases 4 and 5.

- Travel measures include distribution of health alert notices, screening of inbound and outbound travellers, isolation of ill travellers and quarantine of exposed travellers, travel advisories, and possibly border closures.

- In communities, there may be containment measures to slow down the spread of the virus. In Phases 4 and 5, these will be aimed initially at individuals. As the pandemic becomes more widespread, they may involve the general population.

- Legal powers exist at the federal and provincial level to enforce isolation and quarantine measures, but public health officials will rely largely on people's understanding of the issues and on their cooperation.

Containment Measures in the Town of Alliance, Alberta, 1918

"They also have a notice that all churches, schools, shows, poolrooms, and public gatherings will be closed for now, and also no person can enter or leave Alliance by train until further notice,"
—Phyllis

"When my dad went in to meet the train, he says that they had guards at every approach into Alliance and so . . . all the country people were not allowed to come in and I think not allowed to go out either."
—Another resident

"There were no funerals. There were too many . . . you know, the whole neighbourhood was sick."
—Elsie

From CBC's "Surviving 'The Spanish Lady,'"
broadcast April 10, 2003

TRAVEL MEASURES

When individuals and governments face the onset of a pandemic, there will be an intuitive appeal and some good reasons to limit the movement of people across borders, and even the movement and freedoms of people within their own countries and communities. People's first instincts will be to avoid contact with those who have influenza. Out of this sentiment may come an impulsive sense that we should "close the borders" and "keep the sick people away!" Travel measures and community containment measures will certainly be used, but we should not implement them in a reflexive and unconsidered way. They must be used quickly and effectively, but with sound reasoning and careful consideration. Travel measures are a daunting proposition: in Canada, over 18 million persons enter our country annually by air, with 91% arriving at six international airports. A similar number depart yearly from our international airports. Our open land border with the United States is crossed over 100 million times each year, in both directions.[1]

Travel measures and community containment measures have human, economic, and societal costs. Also, it must be understood that these measures are very unlikely to stop a pandemic; rather, their goals will be to slow a pandemic and reduce its damaging effects. The costs of these measures will need to be weighed against their expected benefits. There won't be a one-size-fits all measure to take; rather, the specific choice of measures in the midst of a pandemic will depend upon the phase and other issues.

What Will We Do? What Won't We Do?

It is likely, although not certain, that the pandemic virus will originate outside of Canada. The main usefulness of travel measures is in Phases 4 and 5, and at that point public health officials here may consider international measures for inbound travellers. The use of such action will depend upon how many pandemic influenza cases there are in what parts of the world, and the extent to which human-to-human transmission exists there. Travel measures may have some use very early in Phase 6, or in exceptional circumstances such as in island countries, where they may be more effective.

During Phase 6 of the pandemic of 1918–19, various travel measures were attempted around the world, and none were found to be very effective in slowing or stopping the pandemic. People were travelling largely by rail and ship. With the current extensive use of modern air travel, we expect screening and quarantine of travellers at borders during Phase 6 to be even less effective. If an airline passenger passing through a major international hub like Tokyo, Frankfurt, or Chicago infects a handful of other people who are en route to other destinations around the world with the pandemic strain of influenza, it could span the globe very quickly. No border measures can be depended upon to detect that passenger, who may not even know that she is infected when boarding the plane. No one may know that a novel influenza strain is flying to all continents of the world until it has occurred. Once the pandemic is well under way in Phase 6, most places in the world won't get much benefit from the more invasive and disruptive travel measures. Despite this, fear in the midst of worldwide outbreaks may create political pressures for many countries to use stringent travel measures in Phase 6.

It is believed that "exit measures," applied to ill people who are leaving affected areas, would generally be more useful than "entry measures," applied to people entering unaffected areas. However, unaffected areas will likely have more popular and political motivation to do things like close borders and impose travel restrictions, while affected areas may have their hands full dealing with other pandemic issues. People in affected areas may want to leave, despite any exit restrictions. So it may be that political impulses and people's personal fears and actions run somewhat counter to what is actually most useful on a global scale.

If pandemic influenza starts in Asia, it will probably take up to a month to build up from a handful to around 1,000 cases at its geographical source, and then perhaps two to four weeks to travel from Asia to Canada. SARS taught us, in Toronto, that all it takes is one case of a new infectious disease to enter a city for that city to experience very significant consequences. First we had one case, which grew into clusters of cases. Within days, the face of our hospitals had changed to one of masks and fear. Since it is not expected that massive border screening or quarantine could succeed in keeping every single case of a new strain of pandemic influenza out of a city, experts feel it is unwise to use a massive amount of resources to implement extensive screening or quarantine programs. Those energies would be better spent elsewhere. Before you throw up your hands in despair at travel measures, note that in 1918–19 the world had little realization of what was happening until Phase 6 was well established, and no travel measures were attempted until then. Today our goal is to detect Phases 4 and 5 and to use selected travel measures at that point, when more benefit can be expected.

What can we expect in Canada? We are a geographically large country, with an 8,891-kilometre undefended land border and over 20 million international tourists per year, making it difficult and expensive to implement border and travel measures. Travel measures will probably be implemented when the first cases arrive in Canada, probably in Phases 4 and 5 and possibly early in Phase 6. They will probably not continue when influenza is spreading widely within the country.

Even the most severe use of these measures cannot be expected to prevent a pandemic from arriving in Canada once Phase 6 is under way. However, the judicious use of these measures in Phases 4 and 5 and possibly very early in Phase 6 may slow the arrival and spread of influenza and buy us some time to make other preparations.

Dr. Lee's Perspective
Doctoring for my Neighbours

As one of Ontario's medical officers of health, I'm part of the public health team that watches over half a million people living in Simcoe County and Muskoka, just north of Toronto. These are my neighbours, friends, and colleagues. I also work as an emergency physician at the local hospital, keeping in touch with fevers and coughs in people who come through the hospital doors.

You would think that 14 years of university and clinical training would have fully equipped me for these tasks. In fact, the more I learn, the more I realize that there are great areas of unknown. Walking through the scientific literature about pandemic influenza is like travelling in a forest at night—the trees are solidly there, but the shadows and leaves shift unpredictably, and roots threaten to trip even the most careful traveller. I'm somewhat experienced in controlling infectious disease outbreaks in health care institutions and in my community, but nothing compares to the vastness and unpredictability of an influenza pandemic.

Will it be mild? Will it be devastating? When will it arrive? How will it all play out? No one can say, but nonetheless my job is to make specific recommendations in the face of uncertainty. What should hospitals and individuals stockpile in preparation? When the first of my neighbours falls ill with pandemic influenza, should I quarantine the people he's been in contact with? If someone refuses, there is legal power that I could invoke—but can I justify depriving someone of freedom in order to protect others in my community? Who should have priority access to antivirals and vaccines during a pandemic? How will I feel if I make the best possible decision at one point in time, and later the emergence of further science and knowledge makes me wish I had done something slightly different?

The Canadian Pandemic Influenza Plan

"The Canadian plan is considered by us at WHO as a model, because it has all the components a pandemic plan should have," says Dr. Otavio Oliva, senior WHO adviser. Canada's plan has been evolving since 1988; the initial version was released to the public in 2004. Because of the growing body of science in pandemic influenza and the continued need for detailed planning, there are periodic updates to this document.

Who wrote it?

The plan is developed by the Pandemic Influenza Committee of the Public Health Agency of Canada. Those involved in its development have expertise in:

• infectious disease
• public health
• emergency response
• epidemiology
• laboratory diagnostics

What are its goals?

• minimize serious illness

- minimize overall number of deaths
- minimize societal disruption among Canadians

What's in the plan?

- disease surveillance
- public health measures
- vaccine development, production, and use
- emergency response, health services
- antiviral medication use strategies
- roles and responsibilities of all levels of government to ensure appropriate coordination

Do we actually have vaccines and other tools?

- 10-year pandemic and seasonal influenza vaccine contract with ID Biomedical, signed in 2001
- $34-million contract to develop and test a mock pandemic influenza vaccine, signed in 2005
- 35 million doses of Tamiflu stockpiled at various levels of government, with stockpiling ongoing

The Public Health Agency of Canada has strong links with international disease surveillance networks, including the Global Public Health Intelligence Network. To manage an emergency, it has an emergency operations centre. Each province and territory in Canada also has its own detailed plan, as health in Canada is largely a provincial responsibility, and many decisions will need to take place at a local level. Much of the day-to-day front-line work during a pandemic will be done by local public health workers, essential service workers, and health care providers.

Source: http://depts.washington.edu/einet/doclib/canada.ppt
Presentation by Dr. Paul Gully, Deputy Chief Public Health Officer, Public Health Agency of Canada, Ottawa, January 19, 2006, and http://www.phac-aspc.gc.ca/influenza/pandemic_qa_e.html#toc

Some Travel Measures to Be Considered

Travel health alert notices: Notices distributed to travellers. These should be used, because there's little cost and information is valuable.

The WHO recommends giving information to travellers regarding pandemic influenza symptoms and how and where to seek medical care if these symptoms occur. The WHO recommends doing this at international borders and also at the entry or exit points of affected areas once there are outbreaks of a novel influenza strain. If you flew across a border during the 2003 SARS outbreak, you may have received one of the 31 million health alert notices distributed to international travellers in a number of countries.[2] In mainland China, the distribution of 450,000 notices resulted in the detection of 4 SARS cases, and in Thailand 1 million notices detected 24 cases.[3] This measure costs relatively little and does not interfere with people's personal liberty. We strongly believe that nothing is more important to you during a pandemic than timely and accurate information, which may assist you in obtaining appropriate treatment and may prevent unnecessary spread of infection.

Screening for illness: Travellers could be screened for fever and respiratory symptoms through a self-administered questionnaire, body temperature-sensing devices, or monitoring and interviewing by health care workers. Exit screening applied to people leaving an affected area may be useful in Phases 4 and 5.

Screening is very different from border closures. Screening involves systematic attempts to detect people who might be suffering from influenza. If detected, they may be isolated and prevented from travelling across borders. Screening allows most people to cross borders and accepts that some people might cross borders while an infection is incubating within their bodies and before they develop any symptoms.

The WHO recommends consideration of exit screening from affected countries during Phases 4 and 5. Exiting travellers should fill out symptom questionnaires and may have their temperature checked. Ill persons should be encouraged to defer travel, and if people develop symptoms while travelling they should be isolated from other travellers if possible. On international vessels leaving affected areas, travellers should be offered masks. The WHO is coordinating with international airlines to be able to implement these measures in a standardized fashion.

In Canada, public health officials have concluded that entry screening at borders for SARS during the 2003 outbreak was not successful or cost-effective.[1] The data from four Asian locations and Canada indicated that body temperature-sensing devices did not detect a single case of SARS in the screening of over 35 million entering travellers.[2] Arrival screening, applied to people entering an unaffected area, is not generally recommended but is likely to happen anyway in some places. There's less scientific evidence that it's useful.

Identification and isolation of ill travellers and quarantine of contacts: If an ill traveller from an airplane or other vessel is suspected to be infected with a novel influenza subtype, the traveller may be isolated and transferred to an appropriate medical facility. The other passengers who may have been in contact with the ill traveller may be quarantined. This is possibly useful only in Phases 4 and 5, or maybe very early in Phase 6.

If you're on a plane during an influenza pandemic, and it's discovered that someone on the plane has influenza, you might be quarantined. Transmission of seasonal influenza has occurred on airplanes.[4] After one flight that had a passenger suffering from influenza, and that was grounded for three hours without ventilation, 72% of passengers developed influenza-like illness within 72 hours.[5] On another flight, 15 passengers travelling with an influenza-infected person became ill within a couple of days. All 15 were seated within five rows of the influenza-infected person, including 9 who were seated within two rows.[6] SARS is transmitted in a similar fashion to influenza, and in 2003, on a three-hour flight from Hong Kong to Beijing, a SARS-infected passenger was thought to have infected 22 persons.[7] If an ill traveller carrying the pandemic influenza strain can be identified before disembarking the plane, it might be very useful for this passenger to be met, isolated, and treated by health officials. Other passengers on the plane should be given health information and possibly quarantined, more likely at their homes than in a quarantine facility.

Australia's pandemic plan calls for declarations of health to be made by commercial aircraft commanders: "Positive pratique will be required of aircraft commanders replacing the current pratique by exception. Positive pratique requires the aircraft commander to declare the health of all people on board, whereas current pratique requires the commander only to notify if an ill passenger is on board."[8] This would necessitate standardized training for flight staff and coordination among travel and public health officials. It is not clear how people who are ill with influenza would be identified in a standardized way.

Quarantine of all travellers: All travellers from a pandemic-affected area crossing a border could be quarantined. This is not likely to be routinely used, both because the large number of international travellers would make it expensive and cumbersome and because it would probably deliver little benefit.

What about quarantining everyone coming from a pandemic-stricken area? This has intuitive appeal, but the logistics are staggering. In our era of high-volume air travel, with 1.4 billion air travellers per year and 25 persons per second crossing national borders, it would mean placing tens of millions of people worldwide in quarantine facilities for days, where they must be fed, kept clean and warm, and kept safe from infecting one another. This is unworkable. Remember that an influenza pandemic will not be a brief event but will go on for months or years. Meanwhile, all it takes is for one case to slip through. There are better ways to use public energies and resources.

In past influenza pandemics, quarantine of travellers at international borders did not substantially delay introduction of pandemic influenza into most countries, except in the case of some island countries. Thanks to their lack of land borders and their relative isolation, some island countries had success with mass quarantine during Phase 6 of the 1918–19 pandemic. Starting in October 1918, during the second wave of that pandemic, Australia quarantined ships arriving with a case of influenza for at least seven days. This measure was also applied to all ships from South Africa and New Zealand because of severe disease in those countries. The first cases of pandemic flu were not reported in Australia until January 1919, suggesting that those strict quarantine measures delayed the introduction of the disease by about three months.[2] Madagascar, another island country, had success with the use of border quarantine. It had its first cases in April 1919, while its neighbouring southern African countries already had their first cases between September and December 1918.[2] American Samoa and New Caledonia in the Pacific had similar success.[2]

There were not as many international travellers then, and travel by ship was much slower than by airplane. If someone on a ship was ill, there was time to find out. It was also logistically possible to quarantine people, because they were already on board an obvious quarantine facility—a ship. Most countries, including Canada, are not likely to achieve benefit in Phase 6 from such mass quarantines in our modern circumstances, and should probably not attempt them. In our era of rapid air travel and interdependent economies, it is also questionable whether island countries could achieve the success that they achieved during the 1918–19 pandemic. However, if island countries can tolerate the large costs of such measures, they might attempt them with at least some historical precedent of success.

Travel advisories to limit travel: People may be advised to avoid travel if they are ill, and in some situations to defer non-essential travel, particularly to affected areas. Such voluntary travel advisories are sometimes issued by the WHO on an international basis, as well as by countries for their own citizens. They were used during SARS. There may be some usefulness in Phases 4 and 5, and they are expected to have limited benefit in Phase 6. Deciding whether to use these measures involves a trade-off of costs and benefits.

During Phase 6, travel limitations can be expected to yield a diminished return. The United Kingdom's pandemic plan suggests on the basis of mathematical modelling that a 90% restriction of international air travel might delay the peak of the influenza wave in Britain by one to two weeks.[9] A 99.9% international travel restriction might delay a pandemic wave by two months. Restrictions on travel within the United Kingdom in the order of 60% would delay the peak number of cases in the country by about a week but would have little effect upon the total number of cases.[9] These numbers seem modest given the amount of disruption such actions would entail. On the other hand, even delaying the peak number of cases by a week or two could be valuable in buying time for preparation. The difficult question will be whether it's worth doing, and there's no easy answer. That is a political, economic, and societal question as much as a public health issue, and this will play out in different ways in different parts of the world.

During the 1918–19 pandemic, a number of measures to limit travel within Canada and within Australia were attempted, including police checkpoints and stopping road and rail traffic. These did not prevent or slow down the spread of the virus between Canadian provinces and between Australian states.[2]

Border closures or prohibition of non-essential travel: Some governments may consider closing borders or prohibiting non-essential arrivals from a particular badly affected country or region. This measure would be cumbersome and very disruptive to society and economies. In most places, it would not be useful.

The WHO does not generally recommend a complete closure of international borders or travel prohibitions. It is judged to be excessively resource intensive, hugely economically disruptive, and probably not successful in the end. Closing borders absolutely would mean not allowing the entry of cargo airplanes and ships and barring a country's own citizens who have been abroad for business or holidays. If you were overseas at the start of an influenza pandemic, an absolute border closure would mean you couldn't go home. Absolute border closures would cripple modern economies, and most countries depend upon trade not only for their economies but for food, medications, fuel, and other essential goods. In most places, public energy is better employed doing things that have a better chance of success, such as early detection, treatment, and isolation of the first cases, contact tracing, and community containment measures.

Once again, island countries may be unusual in having some chance of success. If an island country wants to attempt border closures or other restrictive border measures, it must be relatively self-sufficient and willing to accept a huge economic and social cost for weeks, months, or years, and it will have the best chances if it implements such measures early and strictly. This, however, does not guarantee success. Nunavut is effectively our "island nation," because travel to this region is significantly limited by geography and distance, and the number of travellers is usually small. If the government of Nunavut wishes to implement stringent travel restrictions to Nunavut during Phases 4, 5, and even 6 of a pandemic, there might be a case to be made for the possible benefits of doing so.

Revised International Health Regulations

The International Health Regulations are one of only two international legal instruments that are legally binding upon all agreeing WHO member states (the other is the WHO Framework Convention on Tobacco Control). The revised version of the regulations is to be implemented in 2007, but it will probably be fast-tracked, given the current concern over the H5N1 avian influenza outbreak.

What is the purpose of the revised regulations?

• Prevent, protect against, control, and provide a coordinated and effective global public health response to the international spread of disease.

• Minimize the associated public health risks to populations, while avoiding unnecessary interference with global passenger travel and commerce.

• Establish common procedures for public health measures at international air and land borders.

What will these regulations do?

• Ensure delivery of credible, common, and timely disease outbreak information to the public. Too often, false "unconfirmed reports" are quickly delivered by modern news media. Such media reports can harm efforts at containing a disease.

• Require notification to the WHO of all events that may constitute a public health emergency of international concern.

• Set out basic minimum public health capacities for all countries to report and respond to public health emergencies, including implementation of measures such as quarantine at certain international airports, ports, and ground crossings.

• Ensure timely and accurate determination of when an

infectious disease outbreak constitutes a public health emergency of global concern.

- Improve provision of global public health measures and recommendations, including travel advisories.

How are they different from the current regulations?

- The current version, originally enacted in 1969, is outdated and does not reflect today's unprecedented cross-border travel and trade. It requires member countries to report only three diseases: cholera, plague, and yellow fever. It does not take into account new challenges from emerging infectious diseases, such as SARS and Ebola. The new regulations respond to these issues.

How will the new regulations help protect you?

- They will help keep Canada, and other countries you may be travelling to, safer from infectious disease threats.

Source: www.who.int/csr/ihr/en/

COMMUNITY CONTAINMENT MEASURES:
WITHIN A COUNTRY AND WITHIN COMMUNITIES

Containment measures are actions that aim to limit and slow transmission of the virus. These measures can involve individuals or entire communities. In Phases 3, 4, and 5, the web of connections between sick people and their contacts is still small enough that it may be possible to individually identify, treat, isolate, and quarantine people. Sick people and possibly their contacts are likely to be treated with antiviral medications. During Phases 4 and 5, the influenza virus is improving its ability to spread between humans and there are clusters of cases in definable geographic areas. This will allow responses to focus on containing the virus at its source by directing containment measures at individuals in order to slow local and international spread, and possibly even avert a pandemic.

However, in Phase 6, which is a full-blown pandemic that infiltrates many countries, community containment measures become more important. At that point, the web of connections between people becomes so large that there's no point tracing the individual connections. It's more useful to direct actions at reducing and slowing the risk of infection in whole communities.

Containment Measures for Individuals

Containment measures for individuals consist of isolating patients and managing close contacts. Isolation involves sick people: it is the separation and restriction of movement of people who are ill with an infectious disease. The management of close contacts includes one or more of the following: tracing, monitoring, activity and travel restriction, and quarantine. Quarantine involves people who are not sick: it is the separation and restriction of movement of people who are not ill but who are believed to have been exposed to infection. These actions may have differing roles and levels of relevance during different pandemic phases, according to each community's situation.

Ill people: Isolation can occur either at home or in hospital, depending upon both the medical needs of the patient and the conditions of the current pandemic phase. Early in a pandemic, the length of isolation would be the period of communicability or contagiousness, determined largely by our knowledge of seasonal influenza but also by the evolving science about the pandemic strain. The isolation

Dr. Lam's Perspective
The SARS Outbreak in Toronto

In 2003, SARS brought new familiarity with isolation, contact tracing, and quarantine to health care workers and the citizens of Toronto. All patients who entered the hospital had their body temperature checked immediately and were asked a series of questions aimed at detecting whether they might be ill from SARS. Those who had a fever or who provided worrisome answers to the questions were immediately isolated—meaning they were put in a room separate from other people and cared for using specific precautions.

This isolation was imposed immediately, pending a full medical assessment that would determine within several hours whether ongoing isolation was necessary, as well as what other medical treatments were required. Some people who were immediately isolated were judged to not likely have SARS, and so the isolation was discontinued. Others were assessed as being "probable" cases of SARS and strict isolation procedures were continued—including a separate room, the use of protective equipment for health care workers interacting with the patient, and strict guidelines governing the interaction between the sick person and others. Over the next few days, an evaluation was made whether the sick person had a "confirmed" case of SARS.

With a new probable or confirmed case of SARS, contact tracing was undertaken as the next step. This sick person would be asked to identify all the people they had been in close contact with, in order that these people could be contacted by public health workers and instructed to quarantine themselves. Typically, a person's family members, close friends that they had been with, and close coworkers were subjected to quarantine. Quarantine would mean they should stay at home, keep a distance from other people in the home, observe a set of precautions at home, and monitor themselves for any signs of illness. In many instances, one person in a family fell ill, and their family members were quarantined for several days, only to subsequently become sick themselves. In one instance, a whole religious community that was potentially exposed during a funeral ceremony for a SARS victim was quarantined.

During these individually directed quarantines, those who were quarantined were in telephone contact with public health workers, and would receive direction if it was necessary to leave home and receive in-person health care. Working as emergency doctors, we would receive a phone call from either the public health department or the patients themselves to warn us of their arrival and allow us to take even more vigilant precautions.

Now that SARS is gone, we have been left in Toronto with much improved procedures to isolate people with suspicious illnesses. Contact tracing and quarantine are not routinely necessary, but would again be used if there were an outbreak of a worrisome new infectious disease.

period would be five days after symptoms begin for adults and seven days for young children. As the pandemic becomes widespread, the period of isolation at home would be more flexible, probably for the duration of an ill person's symptoms plus an extra 24 hours to be safe. This period would probably be shorter than the five-day standard used earlier on in the pandemic and is based on our knowledge that, in general, someone who is less symptomatic is likely to shed less virus, and therefore is less contagious. Presently, in Phase 3, there are relatively few cases of human infections, which makes it feasible to isolate all the human cases in hospitals. If you are infected in Phase 3, you will be isolated in hospital. In Phases 4 and 5, whether isolation will take place at home or in hospital will depend upon local issues and resources (during the SARS outbreak in 2003, we isolated ill people in hospital). In Phase 6, when there are potentially huge numbers of cases, unless your illness requires hospitalization for specific treatments, you will be asked to isolate yourself at home.

Contacts of ill people: Close contacts are people who live in the same household, have delivered unprotected health care, or have been physically close to an ill person during the infectious period. In contact tracing, public health workers communicate with close contacts and ask if they have symptoms of illness. In contact monitoring, public health workers stay in communication with these contacts, usually by telephone. Close contacts may be advised to restrict their travel or even quarantine themselves completely at home and to take precautions that reduce the chance of infecting other people in their homes.

In most cases, if public health workers ask you to quarantine yourself during a pandemic, it will simply mean that you are asked to stay at home for three days and to stay in communication with public health workers by telephone. The incubation period, which is the time from being infected to showing symptoms of influenza, is usually one to three days in seasonal influenza. The period of contagiousness, when you can give the infection to others, is from about a day before the symptoms begin until five days after you start feeling sick (seven days for young children). Since influenza may be contagious before your symptoms begin, it makes sense to quarantine you even if you feel well. If you are quarantined following an exposure, and do not develop symptoms after the three days, you are not likely to develop influenza from that exposure. Of course, if you develop symptoms of influenza during quarantine, you will be asked to isolate yourself, which is discussed above.

While quarantined, you may be offered antiviral medications as part of a public health strategy to prevent contacts from developing influenza. Tamiflu and Relenza are effective in reducing spread of influenza in households and nursing homes with seasonal influenza cases.[10-16] This is currently thought to be the case for a pandemic strain of influenza. This may be an important strategy during Phases 4 and 5, and possibly during early Phase 6, but it will probably not be a practical public health tool during Phase 6b, when a novel strain of influenza is widespread, because of the large numbers of affected people.

Under "work quarantine," a person can go to work and go home but can't go anywhere else. In some situations, this measure may be applied to health care workers or other essential workers. In the course of their work, health care workers may have a higher risk of being exposed to influenza. Society will need them to work but would also like them to not transmit influenza to others. This strategy was used in some instances during SARS, in Toronto. For influenza, the goal would also be to prevent essential workers from falling ill, by restricting their movement to work and home only, and thereby avoiding exposure to the pandemic strain of influenza circulating in shopping malls, buses, and other public places.

Containment Measures for Communities

As outbreaks of pandemic influenza escalate within a community, the containment measures may widen to involve the whole community. These measures affect the way daily life proceeds for all occupants of a city or area and are designed to slow the spread of infection within that area. They may include self-isolation, "snow days," "self-shielding," closure of schools and daycares, and restriction of large indoor public gatherings. The most extreme option is widespread community quarantine, or cordon sanitaire.

In Canada, the most likely community-based containment measures to be considered will be self-isolation, closure of schools and daycares, and restriction of large public indoor gatherings. In self-isolation, if you become ill with a fever and symptoms consistent with influenza, and even though it may not be certain that you are infected with influenza, you will be encouraged to stay home so as not to infect others in the community. The closure of schools and daycares may be important because children efficiently transmit influenza virus from one to another and then bring it back to their families. This was observed in the 1957–58 pandemic. The other likely measure would be cancellation of large public indoor gatherings, where large numbers of people gather in a small, closed area. Activities that could be affected might include hockey games in an indoor arena, concerts, and swimming at public pools.

The U.S. pandemic plan also describes "snow days" and "self-shielding." These scientifically unproven but potentially useful measures are a more aggressive approach to containing and slowing the spread of the virus. During "snow days," everyone would be asked to stay at home, as during a major snowstorm. All schools and businesses would be closed. The American plan suggests that snow days would be instituted for an initial 10-day period. Anyone who has been infected with influenza should develop symptoms during that period without transmitting it to anyone outside their home, thereby slowing the spread of influenza in a community. Depending upon the new virus's incubation period and period of contagiousness, the period of snow days could be made longer or shorter. During snow days, your household would need a sufficient stockpile of food and other provisions. Emergency and essential workers would continue to work.

"Self-shielding" would simply permit people to decide to stay at home instead of going to school or work if they wished to, even without a generally implemented "snow day." Employers would have to support this measure in order for it to be a practical option for people.

In only the most extreme situations, health officials may use a community-wide quarantine, or cordon sanitaire, which is the most stringent and restrictive containment measure available. The term is French for "sanitary barrier." (Strictly speaking, calling a cordon sanitaire a community-wide quarantine is a misuse of the word "quarantine," since quarantine more correctly refers to non-ill persons.) A cordon sanitaire involves all members of a community, both ill and non-ill. It restricts travel in or out of the involved community, defined by some geographical border. A cordon sanitaire may be legally enforceable on all community members. Only authorized persons, such as health care workers and essential workers, might be given permission to breach that border. It is highly unlikely that this measure would be used during a pandemic, as it is unlikely to be more effective than snow days.

Legal Issues

Ideally, containment requests will be made by public health officials, and people will cooperate. Voluntary action has been shown to be the most effective and efficient method, and it is more humane. Legislation exists to enforce such measures as a last resort, when cooperative efforts are exhausted and the benefits to the health of the public outweigh personal liberties.

If absolutely necessary, Canadian federal and provincial legislation allows the mandatory isolation and quarantine of people in order to protect the health of the public. In Canada, the Quarantine Act allows for a maximum quarantine period of 10 days at international entry points.[17] Similar authorization in the United States under section 361 of the Public Health Service Act and Executive Order 13375 allows the Centers for Disease Control (CDC) and Prevention to quarantine persons to prevent the introduction, transmission, or spread of "influenza caused by novel or reemergent influenza viruses that are causing, or have the potential to cause, a pandemic."[18] With respect to isolation, each North American province or state has relevant public health legislation to compel persons with certain infectious diseases, including pandemic influenza, to comply with isolation, in order to decrease the risk to the public. We hope not to have to use those legal measures.

CHAPTER 7

MAKING PREPARATIONS FOR SURVIVING A PANDEMIC

THIS CHAPTER IN ONE PAGE . . .

- In the worst-case scenario of a pandemic like the one in 1918–19, you would have more than a 95% chance of surviving. If 1957–58 or 1968–69 replayed itself, you would have more than a 99% chance of surviving the next pandemic.
- Educate yourself—it's the most valuable thing you can do.
- Get a flu shot.
- If you travel to places where H5N1 is currently affecting birds, take a few simple precautions if interacting with birds and poultry.
- Adopt healthy habits: eat well, exercise regularly, don't smoke, drink in moderation, and don't contract preventable infectious diseases. It's what your mom told you to do, and it could help you during a pandemic.
- Stockpile some emergency supplies such as food, regular medications, and other essential supplies to prepare not only for a pandemic but for other surprises, such as a blackout, ice storm, or earthquake.
- Buy locally produced food.
- Ride a bicycle.
- Know your neighbours.
- Keep a balanced perspective. Be informed and aware, not panicked.

"What do you mean, I've already survived two pandemics?"
—A patient of Dr. Lam's in 2006, who was exposed
to chickens while travelling abroad

LEARN ABOUT INFLUENZA AND UNDERSTAND
THAT YOU WILL PROBABLY SURVIVE

Even if you had never heard of influenza and had never picked up this book, you would probably survive a pandemic. Consider the worst pandemic of the 20th century, that of 1918–19. Estimates of the numbers who died fall between about 40 million and 100 million worldwide.[1] The other two pandemics of that century, causing 2 million and 1 million deaths worldwide, were far less destructive. Nonetheless, let's examine numbers from the scenario that people fear: one similar to 1918–19. Somewhere between 2.2% and 5.6% of the people living in the world at that time died, mostly during about 12 weeks in the fall of 1918. An equivalent death rate today, with a world population of about 6.3 billion, would mean between 140 million and 350 million people dead. This would be a horrific catastrophe. However, even if this obviously terrible turn of events occurs, any individual person's chance of survival remains much greater than his or her chance of dying. A recurrence of the events of 1918–19 using the most pessimistic numbers possible would give you roughly a 95% chance of being alive at the end of it. If 1957–58 or 1968–69 replayed itself, you would have a greater than 99% chance of surviving the pandemic. In fact, if you were born before 1957, you've already survived two worldwide influenza pandemics, albeit mild ones.

It's all about probabilities. During the next pandemic, some will die and most won't. Nothing can be done to guarantee survival. Before you picked up this book, you probably had at least a 95% chance of surviving the pandemic, and your odds are probably even better, because that number draws from the worst pandemic of the 20th century, a scenario that may not recur. That number also doesn't account for the bene fits of modern public health and medical intervention. Of course, you may understandably take the view that the odds you want are the best odds possible. If that is your sentiment, your goal should be to stack the probabilities in your favour.

Before a pandemic, you should do things that are sensible in your regular life outside of a pandemic and that can help you weather any sort of catastrophe— influenza pandemic or otherwise. Influenza pandemics are believed to be inevitable, but they may not come next year or in the next five years. The things that you do to prepare for a pandemic should make sense even if you never live to see one.

Learn and think about it now. Once a pandemic starts, it will be valuable to understand some principles about influenza in order to assess a complex and rapidly evolving situation that will probably affect your life in some way. Conceptual knowledge and broad perspective will have concrete benefits for your personal decision-making during an actual pandemic.

Dr. Lam's Perspective
Go on a Canoe Trip

If you want to prepare for a pandemic, or for any other disaster, think about the first time you went on a canoe trip. If you've never been, go on one. The tasks of a canoe trip are basic, and so are its lessons. The idea is to paddle and portage from one place to another, find shelter, make food, and enjoy the scenery. One lesson is that things don't happen exactly the way they always do in your regular life, or even the way you expect them to happen while canoeing. That can be all right. While portaging, you may sink into a bog and fill your boot with mud. While paddling, you may go the wrong way and end up in an unexpected (though hopefully scenic) part of the lake. You may accidentally light your dinner on fire. All these occurrences can be dealt with. Dry out your boot, consult your map, and scrape the burnt bits off your dinner. An unusual event like a pandemic is similar: things may not proceed in their usual fashion, but that in itself is probably no cause for panic. Many people may be sick. Most will recover. Everyone still needs to eat, drink, and wash their hands.

The first time you went on a canoe trip, you probably went with someone who knew how to do things like rescue people who fall out of canoes and tie up food high in a tree to keep it away from bears. A pandemic is the same way. Some people spend their entire careers studying public health and infectious disease so that they can tell you what to do when something like an influenza pandemic arrives. What they tell you may not be perfect, but it's a good bet that it'll help you. If you don't believe me, just try to get back into a canoe after falling out without someone telling you how to do it.

Another lesson of camping is that you should prepare for your trip so that really dangerous things are less likely to turn out very badly. There will always be bears in the woods, which doesn't mean you shouldn't go canoeing; it just means that you should know something about bears. Wear good boots so you're less likely to break your ankle when you go over. Know which part of the lake drains into a waterfall so that you don't get lost heading in that direction. Don't cook your dinner inside your tent. During a pandemic or another troublesome time, life may throw you a few twists and turns. Having some things prepared—a closet of food, a flu shot in your arm, and some basic supplies—is just common sense. A bear may decide to investigate your campsite, and you may catch influenza, and since you can't entirely control whether this happens, it's not a bad idea to consider what you will do with a bear in your campsite, or a fever and a cough during a pandemic.

WHAT YOU SHOULD DO BEFORE A PANDEMIC
Don't Cut Off Your Right Arm

Here is our perspective on what to actually do, apart from learning and understanding the issues and risks, prior to a pandemic: if someone could promise you that amputating your right arm would halve your chance of dying during a pandemic, we would still not recommend amputating your right arm. After all, there are a lot of things you need to do with your right arm. Even if you did opt to lose your right arm in order to halve your chance of dying from a pandemic, using our worst-case scenario numbers, you would really only be increasing your chance of survival from, say, 95% to 97.5% or so. We'd rather have our right arms.

On the other hand, if someone could promise you that drinking at least three glasses of water a day could increase your chance of surviving a pandemic by 0.5%— say, from 95% to 95.5%—we would say to go ahead. Why? Well, because it's probably a good idea to drink at least three glasses of water a day anyhow, and it costs you nothing. If you can do things that improve your odds and are probably helpful in day-to-day life or at least are not harmful, then why not?

Of course, no one is going to amputate your right arm in exchange for better pandemic odds, nor is copious daily water-drinking prior to a pandemic likely to make any difference. What is the pandemic equivalent? Someone might suggest that if you could build an airtight bubble in which to live for years in an entirely self-sustained manner without having any contact with the outside world, seal yourself in there before the start of an influenza pandemic, and stay there through a pandemic until either an effective pandemic influenza vaccine was developed or the pandemic was over, you could almost guarantee survival to the end of a pandemic. (Although if there was no vaccine at the end of the pandemic, upon emergence from your hypothetical bubble you might still be infected and develop influenza.) This would be a ridiculous exercise. Not only would it be virtually impossible to successfully achieve such a hermetically sealed state of isolation for the years that a pandemic might take to develop and the several years over which it is expected to run its course, but no one knows when the pandemic will arrive, and the resources that would be wasted on such a project would be far better used elsewhere. This would be the pandemic equivalent of cutting off your right arm—a ludicrous project with no guarantee of success.

We think that people should do things that, in addition to preparing them for a pandemic, make sense in their lives and better prepare them for other crises. These other crises may be other types of natural disasters like earthquakes, hurricanes, power blackouts, unpredictable events like 9/11, or personal crises. We should focus on the pandemic influenza preparedness equivalent of drinking three glasses of water a day.

Get a Flu Shot and, if you need it, the Pneumovax Vaccine
Each year a vaccine is developed to provide protection against the three strains of seasonal influenza that are expected to circulate most widely in human beings. These seasonal strains of influenza are different from whatever strain will eventually cause the influenza pandemic, and the annual flu shot isn't targeted to protect you against the influenza pandemic. We can hypothesize, however, that there may be a chance that the pandemic strain of influenza will share some features with one of these annual strains, particularly if a genetic shift in one of these strains is the event that gives rise to a pandemic strain of influenza. If this happens, then having been exposed through vaccination, at some point in your life, to a strain that shares some molecular features with the pandemic strain of influenza might provide some partial protection. This may mean that the more influenza strains that your body learns to recognize through successive annual flu shots the more chance you may have of partial protection against the next flu pandemic. It is recommended that people who are in contact with birds should receive seasonal influenza vaccines to reduce the probability that they will have a seasonal influenza infection that could allow a genetic shift event to happen if they are simultaneously infected by an avian strain of influenza.

What we know the seasonal influenza shot will protect you against is seasonal influenza. Seasonal influenza is not just a cold, and it has the potential to cause serious illness and death. In a way, it doesn't make sense to be concerned only about pandemic influenza and not seasonal influenza. Pandemic influenza causes higher than average severity of illness and death, but it happens only every few decades. Seasonal influenza causes a more predictable range of illness and death, and it comes every year. If you're worried about walking across a busy avenue once a month, it also makes sense to have some concern about crossing a normally quiet street in front of your home 10 times a day.

The adult pneumococcal vaccine is a one-time shot that protects against the *Streptococcus pneumoniae* bacterium, which can cause pneumonia. This vaccine is recommended for people over 65 and people with certain ongoing medical conditions. Discuss this vaccination with your doctor. If this vaccination is recommended for you, get it. During a pandemic, it will reduce your chance of experiencing both viral and bacterial illness at the same time. In any influenza virus infection, there is a chance of a bacterial infection taking advantage of a person's weakened state, and this can be caused by *Streptococcus pneumoniae.* Even if a pandemic doesn't arrive in your lifetime, you will have good protection against streptococcal pneumonia.

When individual people receive vaccines, they increase the market for vaccine production, and therefore increase vaccine production capacity. Greater production capacity means that during a pandemic, once an effective vaccine is developed, more people will get it sooner. This production capacity cannot be instantly scaled up in the face of a pandemic, so creating additional market demand and capacity in the long term is necessary. We expect that a vaccine against the pandemic strain of influenza will require two doses one month apart to create adequate immunity. Currently, worldwide production capacity of influenza vaccine is in the neighbourhood of 1 billion doses a year.[2] We have almost 6.5 billion people on earth. At the current rate it would take 13 years to produce enough vaccine for everyone on earth, and vaccine production probably won't start for at least several months after the start of a pandemic. In other words, if current vaccine production capacity were unchanged, even once an effective vaccine comes into existence, most people on earth wouldn't get it during the course of the pandemic. It is unfortunately easy to predict that poor countries and countries without domestic capacity to produce vaccine would come last.

Vaccines are a possible direction-changing response to an influenza pandemic. The seasonal influenza and pneumococcal immunizations have excellent safety and effectiveness profiles. These immunizations are like drinking three glasses of water—they're good for you whether a pandemic comes or not. When a pandemic comes, you'll be glad that you had them for their protection from other respiratory infections, and we'd be glad for any other partial and speculative benefits that they might offer. At the same time, vaccines require sufficient production capacity and an effective distribution network. Receiving the annual influenza vaccination increases the production and distribution capacity of the immunization system, which is crucial to the usefulness of any influenza vaccine during a pandemic.

Getting Your Shots

In light of the sometimes suspicious attitudes toward vaccinations in some quarters, we feel it necessary to comment that neither of the authors of this book is in the employ of any vaccine manufacturer. We're not in their pocket, but we are telling you to go out and get your shots. Although vaccines are much maligned in some circles, it is widely accepted by modern medicine and public health that they have changed the face of worldwide infectious disease.

Smallpox killed hundreds of millions of people before its eradication by vaccination. Polio's crippling effects are now limited to only a few countries, and this illness is close to worldwide eradication. Many of the current challenges in vaccination are those of the production and distribution networks. Despite the existence of an effective measles vaccine, and although measles is almost unknown in rich countries, there are still about half a million deaths yearly (mainly of children) in poor countries where access to childhood vaccinations is still a huge challenge.[3]

TRAVELLING TO H5N1-AFFECTED COUNTRIES

If you do find yourself travelling to an H5N1-affected country during Phase 3, which is where we are at the time of this writing, some simple precautions will minimize your risk of contracting this infection. In Phases 4 and 5, it is likely that travel advisories will be issued by the WHO, and by individual countries for their citizens, and you should keep up to date on these advisories and their recommendations if you are travelling. In Phase 6, there are likely to be infections caused by the novel strain of influenza both where you live and where you plan to travel, so the same precautions would apply to both places. At present, H5N1 is affecting mainly birds. The list of countries where it exists grows regularly, so check the WHO website at www.who.int before you travel.

Avoid unnecessary contact with domestic poultry and wild birds. Transmission occurs via close contact with them and with their secretions and feces. Ensure that the poultry you are eating is thoroughly cooked and definitely not pink. Even though there has been no evidence that transmission of influenza can occur from eating infected meat, it is wise not to eat undercooked, pink chicken. It also presents risks of salmonella and other diseases. Cook your poultry to at least 74° Celsius. If you handle raw chicken for cooking or other purposes, wash your hands and cooking utensils carefully with soap and water. Take care not to let the juices of the chicken contaminate other foods that you are preparing. Use separate cutlery and cutting boards. Wash your hands carefully after you handle the chicken and before you handle any other foods.

Enjoy the other aspects of your trip. At the time of writing, birds are at most risk of H5N1 infection. Human cases are rare, and only in very unusual instances is there some limited evidence that transmission from one human being to another has occurred. As always, it is a good idea to wash your hands frequently, especially following contact with a sick person and before you eat. Stay abreast of new developments, and of any travel advisories issued by your home country, the country you are visiting, or the WHO. Follow the advice given in travel advisories.

*In a pandemic, we would see potentially 50,000 deaths
in Canada. We see approximately that number of
deaths in every year related to tobacco.*
—Dr. David Butler-Jones, Canada's Chief Public
Health Officer, September 2005, CBC

Exercise Regularly and Eat a Balanced Diet

Regular physical activity and a balanced diet will make
your body more resilient to any challenge, whether that
is a bout of seasonal influenza, pandemic influenza, or
some other illness. It also makes life more enjoyable.

Have Healthy Lungs: Quit Smoking

If you are a smoker, quit. If you have another lung condition, make sure to care for it properly and don't let it
get out of control. The course of any illness is largely
determined by that illness itself, but it is also greatly
influenced by "co-morbidities," meaning whatever else
is wrong with you. If you have diseased lungs or are a
smoker, minor infections like a common cold take
longer to clear and are more likely to become major
infections like pneumonias. Major infections are more
difficult to treat and may require hospital admissions
for supplementary oxygen or breathing life support. If
you have diseased lungs and get influenza, you're more
likely to become seriously ill and die than if you have
healthy lungs.

In caring for patients when there is no pandemic, our
medical care systems in affluent countries try to do the
best things for each individual patient. A disproportionate amount of the care of lung problems is devoted to

smokers, simply because they have a greater share of lung problems. The resources and equipment we have are generally sufficient, and we often deliver intensive care even when it has become almost futile. During a pandemic there may be a shortage of things like supplementary oxygen and ventilators, which are breathing machines for the severely ill. A *New York Times* article by Donald G. McNeil Jr. on March 12, 2006, under the headline "Ventilators may be scarce in event of bird flu pandemic," points out that during a regular seasonal influenza season, approximately 100,000 of the 105,000 ventilators in the United States are being used; it suggests that a worst-case influenza pandemic would require 742,500 ventilators. We can attest to a similarly tight supply of ventilators, very expensive pieces of equipment, in Canadian hospitals.

In the course of a pandemic, difficult choices may have to be made. We may see, for example, certain age groups with worse survival rates. Smokers also have worse odds of surviving. If a pandemic confronts us with more people who need breathing life support than we have equipment and capacity to treat, the question will be whether resources must go to those who have the best odds of surviving. In Canada we have a system in which people have access to care based on their needs instead of their ability to pay. This does not mean that resources are unlimited, and in many parts of the world including ours, a legitimate question may arise of whether access to certain types of care is linked to the probable success of that care.

Mind you, there won't be a sign at the door saying, "If you're a smoker, don't bother coming in," any more than there will be a sign saying, "If you are between X years old and Y years old, just go home." During a pandemic, treatment protocols will be developed to optimize the success of treatment and may also be designed to optimize the effectiveness of resources. To use a fictional example, if it is observed that people who are put on life support and who show some improvement in their physiological parameters by Day 5 tend to recover, while people who don't show an improvement by Day 8 almost universally die, life support may be removed from those who are not improving after Day 8 if someone else needs that machine. If you have damaged lungs, whether from smoking or other lung conditions, you might be less likely to respond to treatment and to be in that group that shows no improvement on Day 8.

We are not proposing that extra ventilators, at approximately $30,000 a piece, are necessarily a crucial missing link in pandemic preparations. Remember, most people who develop influenza will recover on their own from their illness and never need a hospital or a ventilator. However, it is true that a pandemic may force the rationing of resources. So if you're wondering how to improve your odds of surviving a pandemic, it's best to stack the odds such that you're less sick, and less likely to need these things. If you need them they're going to be harder to get, and if you need them, they might be the difference between life and death.

You can't do much about your age. If you have certain lung conditions, you may not be able to make them go away, but you need to focus on controlling them. However, if you smoke, you can quit smoking. Keep yourself healthy now to improve your chances of surviving a pandemic, and also your odds of living a long and enjoyable life even if a pandemic doesn't come in your lifetime.

Listen to Your Mother

Practise safer sex. If you use intravenous drugs, don't share needles, and use clean, sterile ones (or, better yet, stop using intravenous drugs). Don't contract HIV or hepatitis B or C. Enjoy alcohol in moderation, not to excess. Do we sound like your mother? Maybe, but this stuff might actually make a difference to you during a pandemic. HIV and hepatitis B and C can be transmissible through blood, but blood transfusion systems in North America currently have very high levels of testing and safety precautions to prevent these occurrences.

Have a Good Immune System

At the best of times, people living with HIV are at greater risk when they contract other infections, whether viral, bacterial, or fungal. Whatever the effects of a new strain of influenza in HIV-negative people, they can be expected to be more severe in HIV-positive people.

HIV infection is not the only reason that people have compromised immune systems. There's not much you can do if you are destined to have some non-preventable condition that requires immunosuppressive medications, or that will result in the dysfunction and loss of your spleen and, as a consequence, a compromised immune system. We mention HIV because minimizing your risk of HIV infection is something that you can do by practising safer sex and by not sharing needles if you use intravenous drugs.

For many people living with HIV, complete adherence to a tight schedule of antiretroviral medications is crucial for health. In contrast to most other conditions, missing several doses of an HIV medication is not just bad, it can be catastrophic. If an influenza pandemic brings international trade disruptions and strains worldwide pharmaceutical manufacturing capacity, the supply chain of all regular medications and vaccines, including HIV medications, may be threatened.

Have a Good Liver

Avoid infectious hepatitis and excessive alcohol, which can impair liver function. The liver helps detoxify your body, a crucial function during everyday life and one that is even more important during illness.

Canada's safe drinking guidelines recommend no more than 10 alcoholic beverages per week for men, 7 per week for women, and not more than 2 in any one day. If you're not already immunized, there's effective immunization against hepatitis A and B. Hepatitis A can be contracted through contaminated food and water, and hepatitis B spreads through bodily fluids, including blood exposure and sexual contact. You can contract hepatitis C from sharing needles, and much less commonly through sexual exposure. There's no effective vaccine against hepatitis C. In Canada, hepatitis B vaccination is publicly funded and offered to children and adolescents. Hepatitis A vaccination is not publicly funded for everyone, but the Canadian National Advisory Committee on Immunization recommends the vaccine for "anyone who wishes to decrease his or her risk of acquiring Hepatitis A."[4] Speak to your doctor.

Why Are We Telling You This Common-Sense Stuff?

All of this risks sounding trite, but it's important. Human bodies are somewhat like a house of bricks.

When all the little bricks prop one another up, and all of them are solid and well mortared, the house is pretty solid. If the mortar starts cracking and some of the bricks crumble, the house may shift a bit, but it's still a house. But if someone knocks out just enough bricks with a sledgehammer, the whole house will collapse.

Most people can survive most illnesses that attack just one organ system. What happens, however, is that most severe illnesses lead to dysfunction in many organ systems, and if those bricks are sort of crumbled to start with, the house will collapse more quickly. If you want to optimize your chances of surviving pandemic influenza, do the same things that would optimize your chances of surviving any major illness. Safeguard your health.

EMERGENCY SUPPLIES AND PLANNING

> *Emergencies such as a fire, a severe storm, a flood or power outage, often occur without warning. Your best defense in protecting yourself and your family during an emergency is knowing what to do and planning ahead. Discuss your plan with your family.*
> —Ontario Family Emergency Plan[5]

See the box at the end of this chapter for a more extensive list of supplies.

Support Local Food Production

Buy local, and have a household emergency stockpile of food.

A pandemic could quickly disrupt international trade. The 20th century saw an unprecedented rise both in international trade and in the concentration of the production of goods, whether electronics or food. This continues to be possible thanks to the relative ease and affordability of rapidly transporting goods over long distances and distributing them through international commercial networks. International trade gives us the very pleasant option of buying clementines from Morocco in the coldest months of winter, despite living in a temperate climate. It also means that our worldwide food distribution system is highly vulnerable to trade disruptions, which might occur during a pandemic. The concentration of food production is accentuated by urbanization, such that ever-growing groups of urban people have no ability to produce food.

Buying food grown at local sources on a regular basis supports the capacity of people who live close to you to grow food. If you have a garden, grow some food. Locally grown food will be more likely to be available even if there are movement and trade disruptions during a pandemic. Ways to buy local include shopping at farmers' markets, joining local "food box" programs that allow people to buy a share of the production of a local farm, or just checking where the food in the grocery store comes from and choosing products from places close to you. In times of crisis, it is a great advantage to live in a country that is self-sufficient in food. Support the agricultural industry of the place you live by buying local.

Have a Household Food Stockpile

Coupled with supply chain disruptions, there could also be rapid inflation in the prices of food and other goods, and a pandemic could leave some people suddenly without jobs or income. Having a household emergency stockpile of food will allow you to eat even if food is scarce, or if its prices have quadrupled and you've just lost your job, or if you would simply rather not be outside and exposed to lots of other people who might have influenza. Most commercial supply chains operate on a just-in-time delivery system. Grocery stores do not warehouse months of supplies for entire populations. In addition, the actual arrival of a pandemic will spur many people to try to buy a stockpile of food and essentials. At that point, people's increased desire to stockpile food, coupled with potential trade and movement restrictions, may make the possibility of food shortages very real.

A pandemic will probably last for months or even years. It would not be practical to spend months or years staying in your home or to stockpile enough food for years. However, early in a pandemic, while we are collectively becoming accustomed to new ways for public interaction to occur so that the risk of infection is reduced, it may be reasonable to minimize your time in public, especially in crowded situations. A stockpile of food would be useful, so that you don't need to go to the grocery store, especially if it is half emptied of food and filled with anxious people trying to buy it, some of whom have a little bit of a cough.

Have about a month's supply of food in your home. Feel free to have more, if you have lots of storage space and you happen upon some good sales. Remember that it is only in recent times that this might seem peculiar—and only largely in our urbanized, "supplied from somewhere else" societies. In many parts of the world, the notion of having a season's food in the house is, or was, simply common sense. This kind of food supply will also make you better prepared for ice storms, hurricanes, earthquakes, overnight guests, ravenous teenagers, or an unexpected job layoff. The most practical way to have a food stockpile is to purchase a sufficient supply of staples, and then cycle through this supply by eating it and replenishing it to maintain it. That way, you can eat things before they go bad.

Food You Should Have

Have non-perishables of enough variety that they supply a complete and healthy diet, including carbohydrates, fibre, and protein. Have some multivitamins around, in case a winter pandemic interferes with the supply of fresh produce. *The Canada Food Guide* provides some good dietary guidelines. Rice, lentils, and beans are excellent staples in a food stockpile, and together they can form a nutritionally complete diet, if a not very exciting one.

For a stable carbohydrate and fibre supply, we recommend a mix of dried foods such as rice, lentils, pasta, and beans, and prepared canned foods such as precooked stews, beans, or other dishes. The advantage of dried food is that you can store much more nutrition for a given space and weight, since it has no water content. The disadvantage is that most dried foods require water and heat to prepare them. You will need to think about where you will find water and heat in the unlikely event that utility services are disrupted. Couscous, bulgur, and lentils cook especially quickly with little time and heat, but they still require water and some fuel. The advantage of canned foods is that many are ready to eat. You can survive on them even if there is no heat to cook them. Also, if everyone in your household is affected with influenza, everyone may be too exhausted to do much more than open a can of soup. However, canned foods are heavy with water, and for a given amount of nutritional content, they take up a lot of space and weight relative to dried foods. So we recommend a mix of both dried and canned foods.

We also recommend a supply of dried fruit and nuts, a stock of canned fish or other non-perishable protein, and a supply of table salt, sugar, and oral rehydration solutions or powders that can be useful in helping an ill person to stay hydrated. We don't recommend that any refrigerated food be considered part of a food stockpile, because even a relatively brief power outage, as short as a few hours, can cause foods that require refrigeration or freezing to become unsafe for human consumption.

Think about how you're going to cook things. Electrical and gas outages are possible at some point in a pandemic. This makes it worthwhile to think about alternative cooking equipment, such as camp stoves that use portable fuel canisters. If you are going to use a camp stove, be aware that most of them are intended for outdoor use only. Using them indoors is unsafe and may void your home fire insurance policy. If you have a properly installed and maintained wood stove, this is an excellent way to warm a home as well as cook in an emergency situation. Think about how much wood you need to do this when you don't have another cooking source, and stockpile accordingly.

Water

Even when you are perfectly healthy, you need to have good, safe water to sustain your health. First, water is important because although influenza is not water-borne, you don't want to catch something else while you're trying to avoid influenza. Second, minimizing your chances of contracting influenza involves frequent handwashing, which requires a lot of clean water. Third, if you or your family members fall ill with influenza, an important treatment is hydration, which requires safe, clean water.

Lack of access to potable water is one of the main causes for diarrhea, which kills 2.2 million people (mostly children) per year worldwide.[6] Water-borne infectious disease is a very real and continuing problem in large parts of the world, although in many affluent places we have forgotten about this because safe, drinkable water emerges from our taps. Even so, occasional dysfunction in our water treatment systems can occur and can lead to outbreaks of illness. An outbreak of *E. coli* O157 in Walkerton, Ontario, in the year 2000 caused seven deaths among the 2,000 people who fell ill.[7] A cryptosporidium outbreak in Milwaukee, Wisconsin, in 1993 made over 400,000 persons ill and probably contributed to over 100 deaths.[8]

We believe that things would have to get pretty bad before there would be prolonged disruptions in essential utilities, especially the supply of clean water. The Canadian water supply requires a relatively small number of workers and is heavily automated in most places. It is difficult to imagine it being disrupted for more than a day or two. The provision of clean water should and will occupy a high position in most governments' pandemic priorities. However, clean water is such a priority for human health that everyone should have a plan for obtaining clean water in the event of supply disturbances. You can't go a day without clean water.

Even temporary disruptions can be dangerous to human health.

Many people reading this are probably city-dwellers, who rely primarily on clean water emerging from the tap. If you live near a body of water, as many Canadians do, that's an obvious source of water for you in the case of a disruption in your water service, but you will need to be able to treat it. Buy a small, self-contained water purification system, which can easily be found for a reasonable price at camping and boating stores. There are a variety of systems, with costs ranging from a few dollars for a bottle of iodine tablets to thousands of dollars for portable desalination systems and high-flow filters. One question to consider is which system will effectively treat water from the source that you plan to use in the event of an emergency. Another question is how much water a given system can purify before it needs some sort of replacement product. Iodine tablets are effective, cheap, and incredibly portable, but when they're finished, your system no longer works. Ceramic filters typically last for up to about 50,000 litres before replacement. They're also pricey, typically several hundred dollars. An alternative is to boil water before using it, but this requires fuel.

We think it's prudent to have the capacity to treat your own water for a few days. Another option is to have a few days of bottled water around. Hopefully, disruptions in the safety of water will not happen, and if they do happen we suspect that they won't last for more than a couple of days. However, we believe that the health importance of clean water during a pandemic or during any other disaster is of such paramount priority that it's worth erring on the side of caution. Be alert for "boil-water advisories," which are issued when water safety becomes an issue.

Radio

Get a little radio. This is one of those old-fashioned things that people used before DSL Internet and satellite radio. Ideally, get one that can be powered by winding it up, so you won't need batteries. When the pandemic comes, the most valuable thing to have will be up-to-date information, and this is one way to make sure you can hear what's happening, even if the power is out.

Telephone

Have a telephone that does not require AC power but can operate on the phone jack alone. Telephone networks have a separate power supply and an excellent record of continuing to work during disasters that have caused electrical disruptions. Even if the electricity is out, you still will be able to speak with your friends and family and seek health advice over the telephone. If you have a cellphone only, remember that not only will the phone die after its charge runs out, but the networks can be quickly overloaded by large numbers of users.

Manual Can Opener

You will feel very silly if there's a power outage and you can't open your cans because all you have is an electric can opener. You will also feel hungry.

Flashlights, Batteries, Candles, and Matches

It's pretty gloomy when the power is cut and it's dark, and you may fall over things and hurt yourself. Get a flashlight, and either plenty of batteries or a hand-cranked generator or solar-powered battery charger. Candles also provide light, but every power outage seems to be accompanied by house fires caused by candles. Flashlights are safer, and we would recommend them over candles for light. If you do end up using candles, make sure they are out of reach of children, cannot be knocked over by animals, and are well supported on a flat surface away from flammable objects. Never leave flame unattended.

Bicycle

International trade disruptions during a pandemic could threaten fuel supplies and make it difficult for you to get gas for your car; or gas might become very expensive. During an influenza pandemic, you would be well advised to avoid crowded places, including public transit. A bike is a great way to get around without needing fuel, and without having to stand in crowded public transit. Riding one now will help you get regular exercise, which is also important in being prepared for any crisis including a pandemic. Use your bike now, so you have some idea of how it can fit into your daily routine and how to do it safely. Always wear a helmet.

Warmth

If you live in a cold place, have warm clothing. Have a few sets, so that wet things can dry out, and make sure to have enough warm blankets and covers to keep any sick people in your family warm. A lot of modern urban life depends upon heat emerging from radiators and climate control systems. We think it's more likely that there may be some disruptions in power supplies than in water, since these systems are more heavily reliant on fuel availability and transport.

If you have a fireplace and think you may want to use it for warmth during an emergency, clean and maintain it regularly and know how to use it safely. Keep a store of wood and matches. If needed, a candle also provides a small amount of warmth. Avoid setting anything on fire accidentally.

Medications

Anyone who is on regular medications should consider having an extra month's supply on hand at all times. Replenish the stockpile and cycle through it. We know, however, that medicines are expensive, and your physician may have good reasons for not wanting to give you an extra month of certain medications. You will need to discuss this with your physician.

In assessing your medication situation, it is worthwhile to understand two issues. First, find out what the consequences will be in the (hopefully unlikely) event that you can't get those medications for a month. For some medications, the consequences are likely to be less serious than for others. For instance, if you have mildly elevated blood pressure, and you miss a month of medications, it would probably not be a big deal in the short term. On the other hand, if you have had an organ transplant and you need medications to keep your body from rejecting your transplant, a disruption to the supply of these drugs could be a life-or-death issue.

Second, find out what company makes your medications and how far away it is. If your medications are generic and commonly used, they are probably made in many places, and it is more likely that they are made nearby. If, however, your medications are still under patent protection and if they are an unusual treatment for an unusual condition, the supply chain for them may be longer and more vulnerable; these drugs may be produced in another country or overseas.

As part of your routine health maintenance, make sure that your regular immunizations, like the tetanus booster you need every 10 years, are up to date. There is a chance that a pandemic may result in the disruption of the supplies of other vaccines, if production capacity is diverted to producing a pandemic vaccine once it exists. If that is the case, it would be a shame to survive pandemic influenza only to get a cut on your finger and die of tetanus.

We recommend that in addition to securing your personal medications, which would really be an extension of your existing routine, you have a few "comfort" medications on hand to help someone who is sick to feel better, such as acetaminophen, ibuprofen, and Gravol. Have enough to treat several ill people in your home for several weeks. These medications are inexpensive, particularly the generic or "no-name" ones, and can really help in the care of an ill person. This is discussed more fully in chapter 9, "Caring for Others During a Pandemic." We discuss antiviral medications in chapter 12.

Contraceptives

If you are a woman of child-bearing age, or you are a man who may have sex with a woman of child-bearing age, have a supply of contraceptives around. Remember that a pandemic will probably last for a year or two, arriving in successive waves. It may not be the easiest time to have a baby. You may still decide to have a child if that is in your plans, and this is obviously an important decision that has many more variables than whether a pandemic is happening or not. However, it's worthwhile making a conscious decision about whether to have a child, as it always is.

During a pandemic, health care probably won't function as it normally does. Health care settings may become places that present a risk of contracting influenza. This could be problematic if you are pregnant, or if you have a young child who needs health care. Other issues of concern for a parent of a young child are potential disruption of food supplies, potential disruption of the supplies of routine childhood immunizations, and the fact that children are thought to be a prime agent in spreading influenza. It is also worth noting that one of the demographic groups with the highest influenza case fatality rates in the 1918–19 pandemic was pregnant women. Studies from that pandemic estimated that the death rates for pregnant women who were hospitalized for influenza ranged from 23% to 71%.[1] The reasons for this are not clear. It was not observed in the other two 20th-century pandemics, and we cannot predict whether this phenomenon will occur again, but it is worth having this information, and having contraceptives around during a pandemic so that you can make a conscious decision whether to conceive.

Cash

Just in case there are disruptions in banking services for any reason, it's always nice to have some cash around.

**Masks, Gloves, and Alcohol-Based Hand
Sanitizer or Cleanser**

Have some around. We discuss this more fully in the
next chapter.

DON'T BE TAKEN ADVANTAGE OF BY
"MIRACLE CURE" PROMISES

> *The U.S. Food and Drug Administration (FDA) today
> announced it has warned nine companies to stop selling unli-
> censed products advertised as remedies for avian influenza
> and other kinds of flu. The nine firms have been marketing
> products with unproven claims that they treat or prevent
> avian or other types of flu, the FDA said in a news release.
> Eight products are termed "dietary supplements" and claim to
> prevent or treat the flu or kill the virus.*
> —Center for Infectious Disease Research and
> Policy News, December 13, 2005[9]

Unfortunately, every threat to human health will be
met by an enthusiastic group of entrepreneurs who are
eager to take advantage of people's fear of the threat
and their willingness to trust in an unproven product.
The pharmaceutical industry is no less eager in its drive
for profit, but at least the standard pharmaceutical
manufacturers are obliged to meet strict standards for
the quality of research and production for their products, and you can access data concerning the exact
parameters of these drugs. The same is not generally
true of producers of "alternative" therapies.

The enthusiastic claims of "miracle cure" purveyors
often lack a sense of balanced perspective; their websites
may discuss the politics of the pharmaceutical industry

more than the efficacy of their proposed treatments. This should be a clue to you that things are not what they seem. Unfortunately, claims for turmeric extract, coconut oil, and colloidal silver—some of the many substances proposed to have benefits in treating bird flu—are simply not accompanied by good scientific evidence. It is possible that there are alternative treatments that merit further scientific investigation, but until this occurs we would caution you against using them. Just as it may be worthwhile to perform further scientific investigation concerning the useful properties of "natural" products, it should also be noted that such products are not exempted from causing side effects in their users. "I consider it a public health hazard when people are lured into using bogus treatments based on deceptive or fraudulent medical claims," noted Dr. Andrew von Eschenbach, the acting FDA commissioner, on December 13, 2005.[9] Buy some practical things, like food, a radio, a water filter, and a bicycle, instead of a "miracle cure."

END-OF-LIFE PLANNING

This is a worthwhile topic for everyone, not because an influenza pandemic is especially likely to kill you but because we will all die of one thing or another. An influenza pandemic could result in your death, but as we've already pointed out at the beginning of this chapter, chances are it won't. Many people don't think about end-of-life planning until later in life, but it is useful for everyone to consider it. As emergency physicians, we can tell you that the timing of death can sometimes be unpredictable.

Buy life insurance if you have dependants, and do so with a large, well-funded insurance provider. In a pandemic, there will probably be more claims than usual, so buy a policy from a solid provider that is likely to pay out your policy if you do happen to die during an influenza pandemic.

Think about what you would want as medical care. If you are young and healthy, you will probably want health care providers to do everything possible. However, if there are specific treatments that you don't want, like blood transfusion or certain types of life support, make sure your family knows this.

HAVE FRIENDS, KNOW YOUR NEIGHBOURS

When a pandemic comes, it may be a time in which people need to turn to one another for support and assistance. If you have friends and family close by, and you know your neighbours, they are more likely to help you if you need it. You will be more likely to know who needs something and could use your help.

In modern Western societies, many of us live in ways that are somewhat socially disjointed. People live in apartments and don't speak to their neighbours. Workers commute for an hour to reach a distant workplace, which may be the main place in which they interact with other members of society. We buy goods in stores where we have never met the salespeople before and will possibly never meet them again. Our close friends may be two time zones away, and our families scattered across a continent.

Get to know the people around you. Cultivate friendships in your neighbourhood. Participate in street barbecues and yard sales. Volunteer in local activities. If you live in the same city as family members, get together once in a while. Knowing the people around you means that in a time of crisis, you will be more likely to trust people, they will be more inclined to trust you, and hopefully you will help one another. The whole episode will be less frightening if you know and trust the people around you. We're not suggesting that you should do all these things while thinking only of pandemic survival. Like all the advice in this chapter, this is good planning for any crisis and is good for you even if you never live to see a day of crisis in your life.

In our non-pandemic hospital work, we see many people in a variety of difficult medical situations. Often, an important difference between people who are able to cope with a particular situation and people who are not able to do so is simply whether they have the help and support of family and friends.

Meanwhile, because life is at once precious, fragile, and wonderful, enjoy every day. Don't let the prospect of an influenza pandemic interfere with that. Remember that there are certain dangers in all of our everyday lives, whether these come from automobiles, environmental pollution, infectious disease, or just plain bad luck. We don't let these issues paralyze us, and a healthy concern about an influenza pandemic does not mean that its dangers should overwhelm you. Put them into perspective, and decide what preparations make sense for you.

Food and Emergency Supplies to Stockpile

SOME FOOD AND NON-PERISHABLES
- Rice, lentils, beans, other grains
- Canned meats, fruits, vegetables, and soups
- Sugar, salt, and pepper
- High-energy, protein, or fruit bars
- Dry cereal or granola
- Peanut butter or nuts
- Dried fruit
- Crackers
- Canned juices
- Bottled water
- Specialized food for infants, elderly people, or persons with medical conditions

SOME MEDICAL AND OTHER EMERGENCY SUPPLIES
- Prescribed medications
- Necessary medical equipment such as glucose test strips and needles for diabetics
- Soap and/or alcohol-based hand sanitizer or cleanser
- "Comfort" medicines such as acetaminophen, ibuprofen, and Gravol
- Thermometer
- Multivitamins
- Contraceptives
- Oral rehydration fluids or powder
- Soap and detergent for clothes and dishes
- Flashlight
- Batteries
- Candles and matches
- Extra fuel for car, portable stove, or wood stove
- Portable radio (preferably windup)

- Manual can opener
- Garbage bags
- Tissues, toilet paper, disposable diapers
- Telephone that does not require an electrical outlet
- Surgical or procedure masks (not expensive N95 masks or respirators) and gloves
- First aid kit
- Cash
- Bicycle
- Extra warm clothing and blankets

Several organizations have more detailed lists of supplies and other information on how to get your family prepared for an emergency. Here are some useful websites.

- **Public Safety and Emergency Preparedness Canada**
  http://www.psepc.gc.ca/prg/em/gds/prepm-en.asp
  and http://www.emergencypreparednessweek.ca/
  PDFs/5steps.pdf
- **Ministry of Health and Long Term Care of Ontario: Emergency Management Unit**
  http://www.health.gov.on.ca/english/providers/
  program/emu/emu_mn.html
- **U.S. Federal Emergency Management Agency**
  http://www.fema.gov/areyouready/

CHAPTER 8

THINGS TO DO IN EVERYDAY LIFE TO LIMIT THE SPREAD OF INFLUENZA

THIS CHAPTER IN ONE PAGE . . .

- Influenza infects your body through your mucous membranes: your nose, mouth, and eyes.

- Good handwashing and good cough and sneeze etiquette are always wise habits to reduce the risk of spreading or contracting any infection, and they are crucial to protecting your health during a pandemic. Be a good example for your children.

- "Social distancing" and trying to stay more than 1 metre away from people will decrease your risk of spreading or contracting influenza during a pandemic.

- Use a mask if you need to be less than 1 metre from a person who is ill with influenza, or if you must be in a crowd during Phase 6 of a pandemic. If you can, it's even better to avoid crowds at this time.

- If you are going to be handling the bodily fluids or secretions of someone who is ill with influenza, wash your hands even more and consider wearing gloves.

- Choosing how to go about your daily life during a pandemic means striking a balance between an activity's risk of exposing you to influenza, and whether that activity is essential for you.

- Cooperate with any containment measures in your community if they are used. They are well understood to be disruptive and therefore won't be used unless they are felt to be important.

The Origin of the Word "Influenza"

Influenza traces back to the stars. The ancients believed that you can tell a great deal about [your] future health by studying the pattern of the stars . . . If you have an evil influence from the stars, you can expect disease . . . and that's what influenza means. Influenza is simply the word "influence," the influence of the stars. Nowadays, we have to stick to the virus theory. If you've got influenza, you are infected with the flu virus. It's not as interesting . . . but it has the advantage of being correct.
—Isaac Asimov, author and scientist, CBC Radio's *Quirks and Quarks*, broadcast February 25, 1976[1]

Personal habits regarding handwashing and cough and sneeze etiquette (also referred to in some places as respiratory hygiene), employed to reduce the risk of contracting pandemic influenza, are very important for everyone in the world during Phase 6 of a pandemic, and have relevance during Phases 4 and 5 if you happen to live somewhere where there are outbreaks of a novel strain of influenza. These measures are, however, good general habits to have at any time, since they reduce your chance of catching or spreading a cold or a case of seasonal influenza. Social distancing and community containment measures are most applicable during Phase 6 of a pandemic. Cooperating with measures such as isolation and quarantine is most relevant in Phases 4 and 5, and then perhaps early in Phase 6. We have divided this chapter into two sections: "Central Issues You Should Know About" and "Other Issues Worth Discussing."

CENTRAL ISSUES YOU SHOULD KNOW ABOUT
INFLUENZA VIRUS TRAVELS IN DROPLETS
AND ENTERS MUCOUS MEMBRANES

In everyday life, influenza virus particles travel in droplets larger than 5 microns in diameter, which are released or "shed" from infected persons when they sneeze, cough, or talk. These are large droplets. This is an important detail, because large droplets do not travel very far. It is thought that they spread no farther than 1 metre, which is the basis of the "less than 1 metre" principle: the distance that people should stay apart to limit the risk of infection. Other types of infections, like tuberculosis and chicken pox, can travel in "aerosols," which means they can be suspended in smaller particles with the ability to travel farther.

> **The "Less Than 1 Metre" Principle**
>
> The "less than 1 metre" principle of the travelling distance of large droplets and the transmission of illness is drawn from good scientific evidence. It comes from studies of the spread of meningococcal disease, a cause of meningitis, in army barracks and classrooms.[2-3] Meningococcal disease spreads in a fashion similar to the way influenza spreads. Early in the 20th century, an outbreak of meningitis in a military camp was controlled when the space between soldiers' beds was increased from 15 centimetres to about 1 metre. In 1982, during a meningitis outbreak in a school in Houston, a distance of less than 1.02 metres between student chairs in the classroom was found to be a risk factor for the spread of meningitis.[3]

To infect you, influenza must enter your body through mucous membranes: your eyes, your nose, or your mouth. The relatively large droplets containing influenza virus can directly infect you if you are less than 1 metre from an infected person. This may happen if an infected person sheds virus while coughing, sneezing, or talking and the virus particles enter your eyes, nose, or mouth. Droplets may also deposit themselves on an object; if you touch this object, you then bring the virus to your own mucous membranes by touching them.

GUARD YOUR MUCOUS MEMBRANES: WASH YOUR HANDS

Handwashing is the single most powerful personal measure that can reduce your chance of contracting influenza during a pandemic.

This is what happens: People with influenza cough, clear their throats, talk, or sneeze on their hands. They open doors and push elevator buttons. They may not realize they're sick, because a person with influenza can be contagious and shedding virus particles one day before any symptoms appear. Influenza virus particles can survive on inanimate objects: up to 48 hours on hard surfaces, up to 12 hours on cloth or tissues.[4] You open a door or push an elevator button in the wake of someone with influenza, you might rub a bit of dust from your eye or scratch your nose. Now, you may have infected yourself with influenza.

During Phase 6 of a pandemic, it is probable that you will touch contaminated objects as you go about your daily life, and this might also occur in earlier phases, especially Phases 4 and 5. In this way, you could catch influenza from another person whom you never saw. It will not be possible for you to control who touches things before you do. What you can control is what comes in contact with your eyes, nose, and mouth. Touching and handling an object is not sufficient to cause you to be infected with influenza. It is the act of bringing your contaminated hands in contact with your mucous membranes that allows your body to be infected with influenza. Be sure to wash your hands thoroughly *before* touching your eyes, nose, or mouth at all times. Improved handwashing rates have been shown to decrease infection rates in hospitals and also in community settings.[5] It is estimated that one out of three people do not wash their hands after using a toilet, so this is an especially important measure when you are out in public, especially if you are about to eat a meal or touch your face.[4-6]

Use Proper Handwashing Technique

When medical students begin the surgical part of their training, they are taught how to wash their hands. Why? Because technique is important. Although you won't need surgical handwashing skills in your everyday life during Phase 6 of a pandemic, you do need good handwashing technique if it is to be effective at limiting the spread of illness. If you wash your hands with poor technique and consider them clean, and then rub your eyes or pick your teeth, this is worse than if you had simply regarded your hands as being contaminated and not touched your face at all. Alcohol-based hand sanitizers (preferably formulated with more than 60% alcohol) are just as effective as soap and water and probably more convenient at times. However, the sanitizers are not effective if your hands are visibly soiled with debris or dirt. Antibacterial products have no everyday advantage over regular soap and water or alcohol-based hand sanitizers.

How to wash your hands with soap and water
• Wet your hands.
• Apply enough soap to create a lather.
• Rub your hands together vigorously for at least 15 seconds, covering and scrubbing all surfaces of the hands and fingers. If your hands are visibly soiled, be sure to rub your hands until this substance is not stuck to your skin.
• Rinse your hands well.
• Dry with a disposable towel. If possible, use the towel to turn off the faucet and open the door of the washroom, then dispose of the towel.
• Avoid using overly hot water, because repeated use of hot water can irritate and cause dry and cracked skin.

How to clean your hands using alcohol-based cleansers
These are especially useful where there isn't running water and soap to wash your hands. If your hands are visibly soiled, an alcohol-based cleanser will not be sufficient, and you really need to use water and soap to get the substance off sooner or later. The alcohol-based cleanser will not get to the skin underneath the soiled area.[6-7]
• Apply a palmful of cleanser into a cupped hand and cover all surfaces.
• Rub your hands together to cover all the surfaces of the hands and fingers, paying attention not to miss between the fingers and the backs of the hands.
• Rub until the hands are dry.

A further tip on sequence of actions if you are carrying a personal container of alcohol-based cleanser:

1) Take it out and squirt the cleanser on your hand.

2. Put the container away, since it's now contaminated by your dirty hand.

3. After you put it away, rub your hands together. Now your hands are clean.

More handwashing tips

- Certain areas of the hands are frequently missed: spaces between fingers, creases of hands, and the backs of the hands. Consciously give these areas extra attention.

- Fingernails: It's difficult to clean under fingernails, especially artificial ones. Trim your fingernails frequently, and don't wear artificial nails.

- Dry, cracked skin: Frequent washing dries and cracks hands. Cracks in the skin may be a route for the transmission of infection. Moisturize after washing. Alcohol-based hand cleansers are less drying to the skin than equally frequent washing with soap and water.

- Jewellery: Skin under rings is difficult to clean properly, allowing viruses to hide out, evading a wash. Minimize wearing hand jewellery during a pandemic. Wearing none is even better.

COUGH AND SNEEZE ETIQUETTE

At some point during a pandemic, you will need to cough or sneeze. Do so in such a way that if you are carrying influenza virus, you reduce the chance of spreading it. Cough and sneeze etiquette is sometimes referred to as respiratory hygiene. Not every cough that you have during a pandemic will be influenza. You may be sneezing or coughing because of a cold or your allergies, but remember that you could at the same time be in the incubation period of influenza and be shedding virus anyway. Cough and sneeze etiquette is a worthwhile courtesy at all times, and even more relevant during an influenza pandemic.

Turn away from the people around you. Don't cough or sneeze on people, and especially not in their faces. Ideally, cough or sneeze into a disposable paper tissue, holding it with your non-dominant hand (if you are right-handed, sneeze into a tissue in your left hand, and vice versa). Immediately throw the tissue away in a garbage can. Regard both hands as potentially contaminated, and wash them both thoroughly as soon as possible. Do not unnecessarily touch or handle any objects with either hand until you have done so.

Simple? Sounds like it. Easier said than done? Yes. Try it. Doing all these things in real life may be challenging. For instance, you may need to sneeze on the subway at rush hour. If you are in a crowded place and can't turn away from everyone, try to cover your nose and mouth as well as possible when you cough or sneeze. Or you may have run out of tissues. If so, cough or sneeze into your bare non-dominant hand, or into your upper shirt sleeve. This piece of clothing, or your bare hand, is now certainly contaminated if you have influenza. After sneezing into your upper sleeve, don't push doors open with your shoulder. If you've coughed into your left hand, use your right hand to open doors.

There is no scientific literature to support using your non-dominant hand to address your sneeze, and then preferring your dominant hand if you need to handle objects before you're able to wash both hands. We just think it makes sense, because you're going to need to use one of your hands. Interestingly, in many cultures, such as in India, the left hand is seen as a contaminated hand and performs "dirty" daily activities; consequently, one never greets another person with that hand. Ideally, after sneezing you shouldn't handle anything but should immediately throw away the tissue and wash both hands fastidiously. In a perfect world, bathrooms would be everywhere, they wouldn't have doors, and all sinks would be motion-activated. Since this isn't the case, and the ideal of not touching anything after you sneeze until you thoroughly wash your hands isn't always going to be possible, we recommend using your dominant and non-dominant hands, as well as your shirt sleeve in the fashion we describe above. Keeping a hand sanitizer in your pocket or purse will also help mitigate the unavailability of bathrooms.

Being Coughed On or Sneezed On

At some point during an influenza pandemic, someone may cough or sneeze near you, or perhaps on you. During Phase 6, this is the pandemic influenza equivalent of having unprotected sex. Avoid it. It would be better if it hadn't happened, but once it has, it's good to know how you might mitigate your risk of contracting influenza and your potential for spreading it further. There is no formal scientific literature in this area, so what follows is our carefully considered opinion based on the best knowledge that exists.

Don't flip out. Don't panic, and don't become hostile toward the person who just coughed or sneezed on you. There's no point. Once it's happened, it's happened. Perhaps the sneezer just has allergies. But you may also have been exposed to influenza. If you have just been exposed but no virus has entered your mucous membranes, you may not yet have contracted influenza.

You could ask the person if he is ill, but this is optional. The answer shouldn't change what you do. Our opinion is that during Phase 6 of a pandemic, you should treat any situation in which someone directly coughs or sneezes on you the same way. If the cough or sneeze reached your hands or belongings, wash them carefully. Be especially sure to give your hands a thorough washing before you touch your own eyes, nose, or mouth. What if someone has coughed or sneezed in your face? First, wash your hands. Then wash your face thoroughly. You may choose to rinse your eyes and mouth. Be sure to wash your hands carefully before touching your face, because if your hands are contaminated, there's no point introducing contamination to your face in your attempt to clean it.

You may consider, in a civilized and nonconfrontational manner, advising the cougher or sneezer to employ cough and sneeze etiquette in the future. Finally, if you have been coughed or sneezed upon, be additionally careful in your own subsequent habits. In this way, if you have been infected, you can hopefully reduce the risk of transmitting the infection to others. Remember, even if you contract influenza, you have a high chance of surviving.

DON'T SHAKE HANDS, DON'T KISS PEOPLE, DON'T SHARE SNACKS

During Phase 6 of a pandemic, greet and interact with people in ways that do not involve direct physical contact. Consider this during Phases 4 and 5. Avoid eating food that someone else has recently handled. When you greet someone, just say hello, or bow slightly if you feel that a touch of formality is in order. During Phase 6 of a pandemic, it's really not sensible to shake the hands of everyone you meet, or to greet all your friends with a peck on each cheek.

This is not an exhaustive list of activities to avoid, so you will need to consider situations individually. For example, eating at buffets is not a good idea, since lots of people use the same serving utensils and take food from common platters. Religious ceremonies that involve drinking from a common cup or eating parts of a commonly handled piece of food should possibly be replaced simply by worshipping without physical contact. Maybe you should avoid contact sports. However, tai chi would pose no problem, nor would cycling or running. Consider the principles we discussed above, take note of activities that involve touching other people, many people handling common objects, or putting food that others have touched in your mouth. If these actions are not essential, don't do them during Phase 6 of a pandemic. Consider avoiding them in Phases 4 and 5, and stay tuned because your local public health authorities may have a timely recommendation on this topic during Phases 4 and 5. They're not directly relevant to pandemic influenza in Phases 1, 2, and 3, although following this advice might reduce your chance of getting a cold or a case of seasonal influenza. During Phases 4, 5, and 6 of a pandemic, if there are certain things that you feel are essential, such as communion or other religious activities, your religious institution may think about how to do these things in a way that reduces the risk of transmitting infection

PERSONAL MEASURES TO LIMIT THE SPREAD OF INFLUENZA

PERSONAL MEASURE	WHEN	LEVEL OF SCIENTIFIC EVIDENCE
Handwashing with soap and water or alcohol-based hand sanitizer	As much as possible and feasible, especially before touching eyes, nose, and mouth	Excellent scientific evidence
Staying 1 metre away from people who are ill	As much as possible and feasible	Good to excellent scientific evidence
Cough and sneeze etiquette	As much as possible and feasible	Inconclusive evidence, but good scientific logic
Masks	1) Within 1 metre of an ill person 2) In crowded places during Phase 6	1) Excellent 2) Inconclusive evidence, but good scientific logic
Gloves	When taking care of an ill person and in contact with an ill person's secretions and excretions	Excellent
Social distancing	Phase 6, and possibly Phases 4 and 5	Some scientific evidence, and good scientific logic
Community public health measures	Phases 4, 5, and 6	Some scientific evidence, and good scientific logic

SOME HOW-TO TIPS

Ensure that soap or sanitizer covers hard-to-reach places such as between fingers and on the back of hands. Keep a small container of hand sanitizer in your pocket or purse. Learn good handwashing techniques. Note that if hands are visibly dirty, alcohol-based hand sanitizers are not as effective.

Influenza-virus-containing droplets generally travel less than 1 metre in coughs and sneezes. Keep your distance from people who are ill to decrease transmission.

Cover your nose and mouth with your hand or tissue when coughing or sneezing, especially if near other people. Do this downwards and/or on your upper sleeve if you do not have a tissue. Wash your hands as soon as possible after.

Consider a good "surgical," "procedure," or "isolation" mask if you must be in a crowded situation. At this time, there is no evidence of the need for an industrial or particulate respirator such as an N95 mask. If you are going into a crowded subway in Phase 6, a mask would be a good idea. For a walk outside in a quiet open park, a mask would not be needed.

If you are caring for an ill person who cannot go to the washroom on her own and you will be in contact with her bodily fluids, gloves are advisable. However, remember to remove and dispose of gloves, and wash your hands immediately after this task, so as not to contaminate yourself or anyone else. Wash your hands even more.

It is a balance between what you need to do versus what you can give up during a pandemic. Do you need to go out and take the crowded subway today? Do you need to shake everyone's hand to greet them?

If implemented, we encourage you to have faith in and to follow public health measures and recommendations such as closing of schools and daycares, and other isolation and quarantine measures. The more people participate in them, the greater chance they have of being effective.

SOCIAL DISTANCING AND THE "1 METRE RULE"

During Phase 6 of a pandemic, try to stay more than 1 metre away from other people. Whether this will be relevant during Phases 4 and 5 will depend on your local situation. The transfer of contaminated droplets directly from one person to another without physical contact occurs through coughing, sneezing, and talking when there is less than 1 metre between people.[3] Keep yourself posted on local public health advice. This is not relevant during Phase 3.

When going about your day during Phase 6, avoid non-essential activities that would put you in close quarters with others. Certain essential tasks may require that you are less than 1 metre from other people. For example, if you are a health care worker, caring for sick people will necessitate that you are closer to others. If you are a police officer, you may have direct contact with people in order to enforce the law. Such essential workers, with unavoidable potential risk exposures, will probably have specific risk-reduction measures for those tasks, such as the wearing of masks, gloves, or goggles.

Otherwise, during Phase 6 avoid crowded bars, busy markets, theatres, sports events, public transit, and basically any non-essential situation in which you will end up being close to other people. If there are essential activities in your life that you can't cut out, think about whether you can do these things differently to minimize the number of times you will be less than 1 metre from another person and to avoid large gatherings of closely packed people.

Some pointers on social interactions during a pandemic

• Don't shake hands or greet people with kisses.

• Don't share water bottles or drinks.

• Don't share cigarettes (you should quit smoking anyhow).

• Don't share snacks.

Thoughts on social distancing

• Work: Can you work from home, perhaps for part of the week, if not the whole week? If you must go to work, as many will need to, can your workplace be structured in a way that reduces the risk of transmitting infection if one worker contracts influenza?

• School: Can more teaching and learning happen through correspondence, independent learning, and online/videoconferencing?

• Social life: Can some aspects of your social life go online? Talk more on the telephone.

• Shopping: Can you use a delivery service? You will still need to take precautions with the delivery person and the goods delivered, but delivery isolates the potential risk into one interaction.

• Banking and business: If you're not using online systems, think about adopting them. (But have some cash, just in case they're not working.)

• Transport: Get a bicycle. An automobile keeps you from interacting closely with anyone, but there is the potential problem of fuel shortages during a pandemic. Public transit and travel in airplanes, trains, and similar vehicles will often put you less than 1 metre away from others. Ideally, live within cycling distance of wherever you need to go, and get a bicycle. It is not dependent upon fuel supplies, and you can easily stay 1 metre away from others. If you do need to take public transit, try to use it during off-peak hours, so that you don't need to be as close to as many people.

IN YOUR HOME

Within the home, you must decide what precautions are practical and sensible to address the potential of one family member passing an influenza infection to another. If one person in a home contracts influenza, there's a good chance that other people will be exposed. They may or may not develop illness, but it is very hard to avoid exposure within a household. Influenza is contagious a day before symptoms appear, and then for five days after the start of symptoms in adults, seven days in children. So by the time your ill family member is known to be ill, you would have ideally needed to start precautions the day before. Since you can't know whether and when someone will bring influenza into the household, the only way to ensure that you have begun stringent precautions before someone develops symptoms is to undertake such precautions for the duration of a pandemic, which we feel is impractical.

If no one in your home feels ill, we don't recommend that you stop hugging your children or sleeping next to your spouse. It just doesn't seem worth it to avoid all contact between healthy family members for the duration of a pandemic, just in case someone does contract influenza. A pandemic wave can last for months, and the whole pandemic may last for years.

If one member of the household falls ill and everyone else still feels perfectly well, it may be worth taking some precautions. If one family member is returning to the household after being away for some time during which they may have been exposed to influenza, it may be especially worthwhile to use the 1-metre rule and other precautions between family members. In these situations, there is a clearly identified source of risk to try to protect other family members from. Watch for current public health information during Phase 6 of the next pandemic, in case there are new time periods of contagiousness for a novel strain of influenza. Even if one assumes that all family members will be exposed to influenza once it has entered the household, there may be value in delaying subsequent illnesses. Those who are sick initially can be cared for by those who are well. Hopefully, those who fall ill first begin to regain strength by the time the other family members become ill, and they can care for the people who fall ill later on. The majority of people who become ill with influenza will recover with good supportive care.

COOPERATE WITH "SNOW DAYS," SCHOOL AND DAYCARE CLOSURES, AND OTHER SOCIAL DISTANCING INITIATIVES

Your government may use community containment measures to reduce transmission of disease during Phase 6 of an influenza pandemic. If this happens, cooperate. If you are asked to stay at home, don't go out for a quick game of softball, and don't have friends over for a midweek barbecue. If schools are closed, amuse your children at home, and don't let them play with their friends. If you're going to end up losing income, remember that it's to protect your health.

Measures like "snow days" and the closure of public venues may happen early in a pandemic. They may be used more extensively in some places than others; they receive a stronger emphasis in the American pandemic plan. They may be used when there is still a small number of cases, and at a time when you may not personally know anyone who has suffered from influenza. Such action will bring complaints because of the ensuing societal and economic disruption, and in this context, it may be tempting to regard the restrictions as an unnecessary overreaction. Keep in mind that such measures are politically perilous, and your government knows that they cause disruption to society, so they are unlikely to be used lightly. If community containment measures such as "snow days" or the closure of public venues happen, your government and public health officials will have thought about them carefully and judged that they are necessary. It may be that data on transmission dynamics collected early in the pandemic suggest a benefit in making everyone stay at home for 10 days. If your government or public health officials want you to stay at home, have some faith, trust them, and do it.

Earlier, in Phases 3, 4, and 5, and possibly in early Phase 6a, you may be asked to isolate or quarantine yourself and to be in individual communication with public health workers. Later in Phase 6, people will simply be asked to voluntarily isolate themselves if they are ill. "Self-shielding" may take the form of a general request that people try to stay at home as much as possible even if they are not ill, in order to minimize their potential exposure to influenza virus. We expect that in countries like Canada and the United States, and we hope in all countries, your cooperation will be met by an equal amount of public support. It's a tough thing to do, but by cooperating with such measures you are protecting yourself, and those around you, giving these public health measures a better chance to slow the pandemic. The more people who participate in these measures, the more chance we all will have of avoiding infection until we can be immunized with an effective vaccine.

OTHER ISSUES WORTH DISCUSSING
GLOVES

At this time, no data support the use of gloves as a personal protective measure in routine daily life, and they have some pitfalls. Gloves are an important part of infection control practices in a health care setting, and data do show that gloves reduce the spread of infection in certain situations in health care. Gloves do not replace handwashing. You may wonder how gloves can be important in health care settings, and yet are not advocated in public daily life. It is because the use of gloves in health care is part of a collection of protective measures used in high-risk situations. It may not be useful outside of these specific parameters.

The meaningful use of gloves in health care has some relevant prerequisites. First, they are useful when health care workers interact directly with people who suffer from an infectious illness, and who pose a high risk for transmitting infection. Gloves are recommended when there will be contact with blood, mucous membranes, non-intact or cut skin, vomit, or feces. In this context, the potential threat is more clearly identified than in general daily life, when one cannot know when one might encounter an asymptomatic but infectious person or touch a contaminated object. To prevent influenza droplet transmission in any setting, gloves are not necessary, but handwashing is essential.

Second, in a health care setting, gloves are part of infection control measures for a specific physical encounter between a health care provider and a potentially infectious patient. The nurse or doctor, before caring for a potentially infectious patient, not only dons gloves but may put on a mask, possibly a gown, and goggles. All these barriers are used for one specific patient interaction and then are discarded or sterilized. This kind of focused attention to a particular source of risk using a variety of infection control tools can be achieved as a disciplined practice in health care situations but is not possible in routine daily life. One cannot go through the day with a full complement of protective equipment that one will change each time one walks into a new room or handles another object.

Third, and most important, in health care, gloves are not considered to be a substitute for the essential activity of handwashing, which is still the cornerstone of infection control. There is a danger that by using gloves in routine daily life, a person might acquire a false sense of security and employ less optimal handwashing. Finally, if the gloves become contaminated and are still being used (remember, they are meant to be single-use and disposable), you could be contaminated by the gloves themselves, while you are under the dangerous and mistaken impression that the gloves are providing protection.

If you are going to use gloves, they would be most useful while taking care of a bedridden sick person as part of a careful attempt at infection control that includes wearing a mask. Meanwhile, you should increase the care with which you wash your hands, and not diminish it because you are using gloves. View gloves as a supplement, but not a substitute for handwashing if you are going to be in close contact with someone who is presumably ill with influenza. Some people may choose to use gloves in their daily lives during a pandemic. We can't say that gloves are useless in everyday life, but there's just no evidence to support their being worthwhile. It's important to be aware of the serious pitfalls to glove use in daily life.

USING OBJECTS INSTEAD OF HANDS

During the SARS outbreak in Toronto, some people developed the practice of pressing elevator buttons with keys, or of turning doorknobs using handkerchiefs. During Phases 4, 5, and 6, creative minds might think of going about their lives with a coat hanger, a hook, or some similar device, in order to pull open doors and push buttons. Some people might push doors open with their shoulders or elbows. No formal recommendation exists to use such measures.

You may choose to do these things, but as with gloves, the potential pitfall is the contamination of the object. Say you push a contaminated elevator button with your key. Your key is now carrying a virus-containing droplet. Now you put your keys in your pocket. They shake around, contaminating one another. Later, to press another elevator button, you retrieve your key chain and carefully choose the key that you have designated to use for elevator buttons. Unfortunately, to do this you must handle the other keys, which are now contaminated with influenza virus, and despite using the key that you have chosen for buttons, your hand is now contaminated. Then you feel that there is a speck of dust in your eye and you go to rub it out of your eye.

The core action that you can take is frequent hand-washing, with special care to wash your hands before touching your own mucous membranes. If you decide to use an object of some kind to manipulate other objects around you like elevator buttons and doors, we cannot say there is evidence to recommend this. What we can say is to beware of the contamination of that object itself. Perhaps carry it in some kind of holster or sheath, so that it is more difficult for this object to contaminate other things that you might be carrying or using. Above all, do not view this as a substitute for handwashing, which remains a central action.

MASKS

"[The pandemic] hasn't reached Alliance yet, but they are showing how to make a mask, giving instructions and it also says if you go outdoors or travel, you must wear a mask."
—Local newspaper in Alliance, Alberta, in 1918[9]

Masks may have a role as part of your personal protective strategy, but both their potential advantages and their limitations must be understood. They are not essential, and universal public mask usage is not advocated in the Canadian or American pandemic plans, even during Phase 6 of a pandemic. Masks are, in large part, a personal choice. There is clearly no reason that anyone should be going about her daily life wearing a mask during Phase 3 (unless she is suffering from a case of the novel strain of influenza, but then during Phase 3 she should be isolated in hospital). Specific situations may have specific issues. For example, if you are boarding an airplane leaving an area affected by a novel strain of influenza during Phase 4 or 5, the WHO does recommend that the airline offer you a mask, because this setting poses particular risks.

As to the scientific evidence, masks are much like gloves. There's no evidence proving that they're widely useful in a general public setting, although they are an important element of infection control in the health care setting. Again, this reflects the reality that any protective measure must be viewed with reference to a particular situation, and as part of an overall protective strategy. During the 1918–19 pandemic, in some places in the United States and Canada, mask use was widely implemented in the general public. In some places it became mandated by law. No clear evidence emerged of it being useful in the general population.

On the other hand, there may be specific situations in which a mask would decrease an individual person's risk of contracting influenza. They are probably more worthwhile than gloves. Although neither is recommended or essential for everyday life, even during a fullblown pandemic, if you were offered either a box of masks or a box of gloves, you should take the masks. Gloves really don't offer anything that cannot be achieved by good, frequent handwashing, which is essential regardless of glove usage. Masks do have the function of covering your mouth and nose—two of the places where you have mucous membranes.

Here's the way you should look at it: If someone told you that you were going to spend some time in a room with a person who has influenza, and you had a choice of either sitting half a metre away wearing the best mask in the world, or sitting 3 metres away without a mask, we think you'd be better off sitting 3 metres away, unmasked. If you had to sit half a metre away from that person with or without a mask, you should take the mask.

When to Use Masks

If you need to be involved in situations or activities that you feel are essential, but in which you might not be able to maintain social distance, these would be times to consider using a mask. For example, if you must attend a crowded religious service during Phase 6 of a pandemic, this would be a strategic time to use a mask. Don't view the mask as a licence to do things that you wouldn't otherwise do. As you are considering boarding the subway or an airplane during a pandemic, ask yourself, "Is this activity so important to me that I would do it during a pandemic even if I didn't have a mask?" If the answer is yes, and you realize that it may not be possible to maintain social distance during this activity, this is the strategic time to use a mask. A mask would be one reasonable way to mitigate the risk of these activities. If the answer is "No, I wouldn't do this without a mask," then don't do it at all.

Use Masks While Caring for People with Influenza

If some people in your household are sick, and some are not, it's reasonable for all family members to wear masks while the non-sick are providing physical care for the sick or coming within 1 metre of them. If some members of your household contract influenza from other people in the house, despite masks and other precautions, it was probably inevitable. Don't be angry with anyone or view it as a failure of the masks or other precautions. Remember, people shed virus before having any symptoms, and influenza is very contagious.

The situation in which it would be most worthwhile for you to use a mask is if you do not have influenza, you are going to enter the home of a family member or friend to care for them, and you will physically assist them, whether this is in eating, moving around, toileting, or bathing. At this point, you are delivering health care within 1 metre of a person with influenza, and here masks have a proven benefit. We will discuss this further in chapter 9, "Caring for Others During a Pandemic." If you are sick with influenza yourself and must go out to seek health care or for some other essential activity, wear a mask to reduce the chance of spreading influenza.

Types of Masks

Get "surgical," "procedural," or "isolation" masks that are comfortable and fit your face well. You don't need N95 or "submicron" masks or industrial respirators, which have better filtration but are more expensive. N95 and submicron masks are hot and stifling, and we can tell you from personal experience that you will have a constant desire to rip them off your face. The wearer of an N95 is much more likely to fiddle with it and try to reposition it, or take it off "just for a second," all of which can lead to its contamination or complete failure as a protective device. In Toronto during SARS, N95 masks became the standard device used in health care settings because it was unclear at the outset how SARS was transmitted; but for most diseases including influenza, they are unnecessary. N95 masks are necessary for much smaller aerosol particles, which occur with tuberculosis, chicken pox, and measles; they are unnecessary for diseases like influenza, since the current scientific evidence indicates that influenza in everyday life is mostly transmitted by large droplets, not by aerosols.

Mask Use Pitfalls

Masks are single-use devices, intended to be used for a few hours. Once they become wet with condensation from breathing, they are less effective. To go through a pandemic wearing fresh masks all the time, one would need thousands of masks. Masks are susceptible to damage. If they have small tears, damage that isn't visible to the naked eye, they no longer provide the same degree of protection, which may result in your feeling an unwarranted sense of safety from wearing a damaged mask. Masks themselves can become contaminated. Then your mask is an object that can contaminate you and that happens to be sitting on your face.

The biggest pitfall would be if a mask reduces your adherence to staying 1 metre away from other people or decreases your attention to the more important activities of handwashing or cough and sneeze etiquette. Those other measures are really still the core actions to reduce one's chance of contracting influenza or spreading it.

Reusing Masks

The best advice is: Don't do it. It's like reusing a condom—obviously a bad idea from both infection control and aesthetic points of view. However, we recognize that during a pandemic, some people may want or need to reuse their masks if there is an insufficient supply. Some people may be taking care of sick family and loved ones, and may simply not be able to get more masks, so reuse may be the only viable strategy. A used mask may be better than none in caring for an ill family member. There is no scientifically based guidance that we can give you on reusing your masks.

However, if you're going to do it anyhow, here's what we think makes sense. Don't share masks. If you are using them in your household, label them so that it is clear whose masks are whose. The influenza virus can survive on objects for some time, so try not to wear a particular mask again until several days after you last wore it. Have a number of masks, so that you can rotate through them in sequence. Disposable masks are not designed to be washed, so don't wash them—after each use, just hang each one up and leave it for a few days. Inspect masks before reusing them and discard any visibly damaged or soiled ones. Understand that reused masks provide substandard protection, so you really shouldn't do anything with such a mask that is not so crucial that you would do it even if you didn't have any mask at all.

CHAPTER 9

CARING FOR OTHERS DURING A PANDEMIC

THIS CHAPTER IN ONE PAGE . . .

- Stay aware of the latest influenza advice. Current information will be given via the Internet, television, radio, and newspapers. In many places, individual medical advice may be offered by public health and government through the telephone and the Internet.

- Most people will have only mild or moderate influenza illness even during a pandemic. They will not require hospitalization but will recover well at home if well cared for. However, don't hesitate to seek medical advice if you are unsure.

- Care for someone with influenza at home by providing fluids, food, and "comfort" medications like acetaminophen (Tylenol/Tempra), ibuprofen (Advil/Motrin), and dimenhydrinate (Gravol). Provide social support and obtain medical help as needed.

- Hydration is crucial. Do everything possible to help an ill person stay hydrated.

- To decrease the risk of transmission from an ill family member to a not-ill member, use handwashing, keep 1 metre away when possible, and practise good cough and sneeze etiquette. You may want to organize your house into "ill" and "not ill" zones.

- Vital signs such as temperature, pulse rate, breathing rate, and urine output can be helpful in giving you an idea how sick a person is, but don't obsess over them or rely on them totally. In caring for someone, trust your instincts and err on the side of caution, especially if you are worried about a person's condition, and get medical advice if needed.

"My brother's coming back from the first Great War and they
had this flu going on very violently at that time . . . And
they had what they called was a soup kitchen for everybody in
those days, and they would bring the food or soup or whatever
and put it at the door, and if you were lucky enough to have
somebody on their feet in the house, they would come of course
and get the soup and bread and try to feed the rest, and I can
truthfully say that I can attribute my life to my sister, because
she and my brother Earl were the only two who could walk."
—1918–19 pandemic survivor Bernice Manning, on
CBC Radio's *The Current*, broadcast June 23, 2005[1]

YOU CAN CARE FOR SOMEONE WITH INFLUENZA

You have the ability to help your family members, friends, and others during an influenza pandemic. During Phases 3, 4, and 5, there will be few enough cases of the novel strain of influenza that everyone with this illness will receive professional medical attention, and probably hospitalization for treatment and isolation. In Phase 6, there will be so many cases of illness that hospital admission will be reserved for those who are significantly ill and need specialized treatments. People with milder illness will need to be cared for at home. Most of what will be needed to care for people with influenza during a pandemic does not require formal health care training. If you care for someone at home, you should know some important things about influenza and understand some basic principles about taking care of people who are ill.

Anecdotal reports from the 1918–19 pandemic describe people in the United States and elsewhere dying while too exhausted to move from bed, while those around them were too weakened by their own illness or terrified to bring them food and water.[2] It is speculated that some people died because no one was either able or willing to help them survive in very basic ways, such as keeping them hydrated. There are accounts of children being orphaned, with no one willing to adopt them because they came from an influenza-affected household. Situations like death by dehydration are often preventable if non-professional people are willing to help.

Stay well informed about what is happening in your community. Listen to the radio and watch the news, but be skeptical of coverage that is either grimly dramatic or unrealistically positive. Pay attention to public health announcements. Medical care systems may operate differently during a pandemic, and there may be an expanded, publicly organized telephone or Internet medical advice service in your community. Use them early, if you are caring for someone with influenza. Some treatments may be effective only if started early. What kind of illness is best served by which treatment, and when it should and can be delivered, will not be precisely known until the pandemic is under way, but issues of timing may be important.

During Phase 6 of a pandemic, medical care systems will be focused. One priority will be treatments that are proven to make a difference. Another priority will be to care for people who are too sick to be cared for by lay people at home. People who are well enough to stay at home will be asked to do so. The majority will recover with home treatment, possibly assisted by medications. Know how to deliver high-quality home care to people who can safely stay at home, and know when to be concerned that a person may need further professional care. Be a confident lay health care provider, but don't put yourself in the awkward position of "playing doctor." If someone is ill, help her. She may not be able to get by without you, and your role is immensely valuable. Meanwhile, seek medical advice by using available telephone and Internet advice services in your community. If you are concerned that someone is seriously ill with influenza, or that his illness has an unusual feature, get a professional opinion as to whether he needs an in-person medical assessment. Don't make decisions that you don't feel comfortable making; err on the side of seeking a professional opinion. Doing this will help an individual person. Caring for someone at home will also help the medical care system, by allowing it to focus its energies on people with severe disease, which will help ensure that hospitalization and more involved care is available if you or your family members need it.

WHAT TO EXPECT IN A PERSON WITH INFLUENZA

A typical case of seasonal influenza begins suddenly and features fever, chills, muscle aches, headache, loss of appetite, and extreme fatigue. A patient often has a cough, sore throat, and congestion. There may be vomiting, diarrhea, and abdominal pain, which are more common in children. The illness may involve delirium or confusion, more commonly in the elderly and in infants. One difficulty is that all these symptoms may also appear with illnesses other than influenza. Lab testing through a swab of the nasal passages can help to confirm the diagnosis of influenza but may not be universally available to doctors and patients. Doctors usually diagnose seasonal influenza by assessing groups of symptoms and knowing how prevalent influenza is in their community. In most cases, major symptoms resolve in a few days, although cough and fatigue often persist for up to two weeks.

Influenza pandemics typically bring an illness with symptoms similar to seasonal influenza, but with some differences. The illnesses in 1957–58 and 1968–69 were very similar to seasonal influenza. The large majority of people made a good recovery with no specific treatment, although a greater than usual proportion of cases involved medical complications, including death. Most of the cases in 1918–19 were also of this pattern, and the large majority of people recovered. A subset of cases progressed quickly and dramatically to death—historical reports tell us of people who died only hours or days after experiencing the first symptoms of influenza, often with a telltale change of skin colour to a blue or black hue, probably indicating that the rapid progression of disease was starving the body of oxygen. A small proportion of people with the 1918–19 strain of influenza experienced profuse, spontaneous bleeding from all of their orifices, and many such individuals died.[2] This was not seen in the other two pandemics of the 20th century, nor is it seen as a feature of seasonal influenza. It may not be a part of the next pandemic.

During Phases 3, 4, and 5, the typical features of a case of influenza caused by the novel virus will be studied. During these phases, all possible cases will probably be investigated with lab testing to confirm diagnosis. Possibly in Phases 4 and 5, and certainly in Phase 6, what is called a "clinical case definition" will be generated, so that people with a defined combination of physical signs and symptoms will be treated on the assumption that they have influenza, without lab test confirmation. During Phase 6, lab testing may not be universally used, as the number of cases would overwhelm the lab testing capacity. Sufficient experience using the clinical case definition will be used to make the diagnosis in each individual.

Our discussion categorizes influenza as mild, moderate, or severe disease. These are not formal medical definitions of severity; instead, we are using a functional perspective that we think is more relevant in this context. For our discussion, people with mild influenza are those who can care for themselves, meaning they can move around, eat, clean themselves, and breathe without difficulty. They are likely to make a good recovery without physical help from others, provided that necessary supplies are available. We describe people with a moderate case of influenza as those who need physical help, such as assistance with eating and cleaning themselves, but who do not have difficulty with swallowing or breathing, or other complications. They can probably do well and recover at home with non-professional help. People with a severe case of influenza are discussed here as those who need intensive professional attention in a health care institution in order to survive.

There are grey zones between these categories. In the course of illness, people get better or worse. This may happen quickly or slowly. Infants and children can usually bounce back more quickly, but they can also deteriorate rapidly; therefore, you should be more cautious with them. Good, non-professional help has a huge role to play in preventing the deterioration from mild to moderate, or from moderate to severe illness. Most people who develop influenza will recover with the assistance of those around them. On the other hand, even with the best attention from loving family members, friends, and the best professional medical intervention available, some people will unfortunately succumb to influenza.

WHAT TO DO FOR SOMEONE WITH INFLUENZA
Mild Influenza

Most people with influenza have fever, sore throat, cough, runny nose, fatigue, headache, muscle weakness, and muscle pain. They may have diarrhea and vomiting. There are similarities to a cold, and there are also important differences. When people get a "head cold," they mostly feel miserable because their noses are stuffy and they are coughing. With a case of influenza, people feel exhausted. Every muscle in their body hurts. Even with a typical, mild case of influenza, movement may require great effort and involve physical pain.

With lots of fluid, rest, and adequate nutrition, most people with influenza will get better in one to two weeks. People with mild influenza are those who can physically care for themselves. You can help by being their supply service and social support. Make sure people with mild influenza have food, fluids, clean clothing, basic over-the-counter "comfort" drugs, and their regularly prescribed medications. People with mild illness can monitor their own temperature and heart rate if they want to. It may not be essential. If they feel that they are drinking well, and urinating as much as usual, this is a reasonable indicator that they are well hydrated. Seek medical advice from publicly organized telephone or Internet channels early during the illness.

Moderate Influenza

In a moderate case of influenza, an ordinary person with no health care training can play a key role in helping someone get better. People with moderate influenza have symptoms similar to those of people with mild influenza, but they are too weak to get their own food, keep themselves clean, and go to the washroom unassisted. They are still able to breathe well and easily, and can swallow enough fluids to keep themselves hydrated. Their thinking and speech is coherent, and they may still make a good recovery at home. They would certainly benefit from an early medical opinion. Remote advice via public health or government telephone or Internet advice would be an appropriate first step. You can be a caregiver. Your priorities are to help them drink lots of fluids, feed them, provide basic medications, ensure they receive prescribed medications, and keep them comfortable, clean, and warm.

Monitor heart rate, breathing rate and effort, and physical condition, so that you know if things are going in the wrong direction. An important issue is hydration. When suffering from influenza, people may need more fluid than usual. Fever increases the loss of fluid through skin, and breathing faster means that more fluid escapes in breath. Diarrhea and vomiting also result in fluid loss. A healthy adult can survive for weeks without eating, but mere days without water. Our body's cells, our blood, and the spaces between our body tissues are all filled with fluid. Insufficient fluid in the body impairs all of the body's functions and eventually leads to death.

To hydrate an ill person who is too weak to feed herself, you may have to spoon-feed her, or give her fluids with a straw. This is labour-intensive but essential. The average adult needs, at minimum, 2.5 to 3 litres of fluid a day. How much fluid is going into someone is a useful piece of information, and a sharp decline from one day to the next is cause for concern. However, because illness changes fluid requirements, and because requirements may differ from person to person, knowing how much is going in is not enough to know that someone is sufficiently hydrated. More important is the overall perspective combining vital signs, dryness of the tongue and other mucous membranes, and urine output.

Hydration by mouth can be just as good as intravenous hydration. As long as someone is able to swallow well, he can stay well hydrated by mouth. Even if a person is vomiting, if he is able to continue drinking fluids, he will probably be able to stay hydrated. The best thing is for such an ill person to constantly sip small amounts of fluids at a time, so that over a 24-hour period he consumes plenty of fluids but is not trying to gulp a litre in one sitting. This is easier for the stomach to handle without becoming upset.

Almost any fluid is fine for someone who is still eating a variety of things, but the less food a person is taking in her diet, the more it may be worthwhile for the fluid to be a specific rehydration solution. If a person has been unable to take food for quite a while or has become dehydrated, and you are actively trying to rehydrate her, try an oral rehydration solution. Buy a prepackaged solution or powder or, as a second option, include some salt and sugar in your stockpile of emergency supplies so you can make a solution using the recipe we have included. If the sick person doesn't like these fluids and won't take them, the next best alternative is to give her whatever fluid she wants. It's better that a person get enough of any reasonable fluid, rather than none of a specific oral rehydration solution.

Severe Influenza

A case of influenza is severe when someone has complications from the infection, or can't get enough oxygen on his own, or can't swallow enough fluids to stay hydrated. He needs an in-person medical assessment, and if the assessment confirms these issues, he probably cannot be adequately cared for at home despite a lay person's best efforts. Someone who cannot get enough oxygen into his body from normal air will need extra oxygen. Someone who cannot swallow enough fluid to stay hydrated will need to receive fluid in some other way. Don't expect yourself to make a final decision as to whether one of these problems exists. If you decide that your loved one is not severely ill, but he is, and then he dies, you will wish you hadn't made that decision yourself. On the other hand, if you become certain that he is severely ill, but he isn't, you may panic unnecessarily and be less able to help him effectively. As a lay care provider, know when to be concerned about severe influenza, and then help this person by seeking professional advice.

Recognize when someone may be having difficulty getting enough oxygen. If a person is breathing fast, or has significantly increased effort, or has difficulty speaking these are signs of lung or oxygen problems. A common complication of influenza is pneumonia. This may be signalled by the above signs or a worsening cough, or simply by a person feeling really lousy. Although it is possible for someone to survive pneumonia at home without specific therapy, developing pneumonia increases a person's chance of dying and would usually be treated with prescription medications. Meanwhile, it is important for the diagnosis of pneumonia to come from a professional assessment, because all medications carry risks of side effects and complications. Someone who had lung problems even before she got influenza still has those lung problems. She is more vulnerable to lung complications of influenza infection, and you should be more vigilant in watching out for breathing problems. Also, whatever puffers or lung medications were routine for her before she got influenza remain important. Make sure that she gets them.

Someone with influenza could become delirious or confused. His speech may not make sense or may become incomprehensible. He may not recognize people that he normally recognizes. This may signal severe dehydration or a wide range of potential issues that need a professional medical assessment.

Recognize when someone can't swallow, which may occur if she becomes more sleepy and less responsive. A person cannot be hydrated by mouth if she cannot swallow properly. If a person coughs persistently when given fluids or food, she may have lost the ability to direct the fluid or food into the stomach, and it may enter the lungs. This is called aspiration. It can cause serious breathing problems and may lead to an especially serious case of pneumonia. Don't feed her. Seek professional help. This should not be an issue in a person who is alert enough to talk and communicate easily, unless she has some other unusual medical problem.

We have yet to meet the virus that will cause the next influenza pandemic. We can't predict everything about the illness it will cause. Remember also that people will still have non-influenza medical problems during an influenza pandemic. Someone with chest pain may still have a heart attack. Someone who is achy all over and has fallen down some stairs may have a broken bone. If you are helping anyone who seems to have some problem that is unusual, get medical advice.

ORGANIZING YOUR HOUSEHOLD WHEN
THERE IS INFLUENZA IN THE HOUSE

If there are ill people and not-ill people in your home, have a zone for those who are ill, and a zone for the not-ill. If you have two bathrooms, designate one bathroom for each zone. If the ill people do not require physical care from the not-ill people, they should stay separate. Have a threshold area between the zones where the ill people can leave things for the not-ill and vice versa, keeping 1 metre apart. If the ill people require physical care from the not-ill people, the care providers should observe extra precautions when entering the zone of the ill people. Handwashing and cough and sneeze etiquette are important for everyone in this situation, and masks will be useful when there is less than 1 metre between the ill and the not-ill. If the care provider is going to be in contact with the bodily fluids or secretions of the ill person, gloves are advisable in addition to handwashing.

If the not-ill people retrieve objects such as dirty dishes or dirty clothes used by the ill from the threshold between the zones, they should treat them as being contaminated, immediately wash them, and then wash their own hands carefully. It's probably fairly obvious that the ill should not be doing laundry or washing dishes that are to be used by the not-ill. Laundry can be washed in a washing machine with warm or cold water and regular detergent. You don't need to separate the laundry of ill and not-ill people. Avoid "hugging" the laundry. Pick it up by using only your hands. Dirty dishes and utensils can be washed either by hand, with regular soap and water, or in a dishwasher. If they are well washed, you don't need a separate set of dishes for the ill and the not-ill. Ill people should place tissues that they have used in a bag, which can be disposed of with other household waste.

Someone else in the home may still end up getting influenza. A person sheds virus for a day before feeling ill, potentially exposing those around him before anyone knows that the influenza virus has entered the house. Influenza is a highly infectious virus, and it's difficult to eliminate every possible way that one person could expose another in the same house. Nonetheless, it's still worthwhile to divide your house into such zones, because it's possible that it will prevent or delay infection. Even if your system eventually slips, delaying infection is useful because if people take turns being sick, they can take turns caring for one another.

Even if you decide not to divide your house into different areas, once there is influenza in your house, you should observe increased handwashing precautions, cough and sneeze etiquette, and social distancing within the home. Communicate, and provide moral support. Talk, trade witty remarks, play charades across the threshold between your zones.

HOW SHOULD I DECIDE WHETHER TO TAKE
THE RISK OF HELPING?

We assume that people will generally care for their close family members. Whether people choose to help neighbours, or friends in other households, will be more of a personal decision. Some ways of helping are less risky than others. If you help someone while maintaining the standard precautions for everyday life during Phase 6 of a pandemic, which include handwashing, cough and sneeze etiquette, and social distancing, helping this person does not really increase your risk of influenza more than any other daily activity. As in the 1918–19 pandemic, leaving prepared food at a sick person's door may in itself be of great assistance.[3]

A person with mild influenza may simply need someone to obtain important supplies for him. He may not have the strength to go out, and it is better for the community if he is not in public where he can potentially infect others. You may help this person a great deal by simply bringing him groceries and other essentials. A person with moderate influenza may need someone to help her eat, clean herself, and use the toilet. If you are going to be less than 1 metre away, or if you need to touch her, you will increase your risk of contracting influenza. You will have to decide if you can accept this increased risk, while taking precautions to minimize the risk. Your risk will be minimized by handwashing, using cough and sneeze etiquette, and using protective measures such as masks when in close proximity. Use gloves if you will be touching an ill person's fluids or secretions.

If a person you know clearly has severe influenza that you can't offer anything useful for, and prompt, professional medical care can definitely be obtained

INFLUENZA: HOW TO HELP SOMEONE, AND HOW

SEVERITY	DESCRIPTION	WHAT TO DO FOR THE PATIENT
Mild	• fever, sore throat, cough, runny nose, fatigue, general weakness, and muscle pain • patient can feed and clean himself	• supply patient with food, plenty of fluids, comfort medications such as acetamino-phen, ibuprofen, and dimenhydrinate (Gravol), as well as prescribed medications • give moral support • obtain medical advice[a] • patient may monitor his own heart rate, temperature, and amount of urination • caregiver should monitor breathing rate and effort
Moderate	• same as above, but patient is too weak to feed and clean himself • patient is able to breathe easily and swallows with no difficulty • patient can talk comfortably	• focus on hydration • feed the patient, clean her, help her be comfortable • administer comfort medications and prescribed medications • obtain medical advice[a] • monitor heart rate, temper-ature, breathing rate and effort, and amount of urination
Severe	• be concerned about the following: 1) patient can't swallow 2) patient isn't getting enough oxygen 3) patient has complications of influenza	• obtain medical advice

a How you obtain medical advice will depend upon how this is happening in your community. The initial assessment may be by telephone or Internet. For mild and moderate influenza, this may be sufficient, and an in-person assessment may not be necessary. Someone who potentially has severe influenza is going to need an in-person medical assessment, but if you make contact by telephone or Internet first, you can receive specific directions regarding where to go and what to do.

TO MINIMIZE YOUR OWN RISK

HOW TO MINIMIZE YOUR OWN RISK

- stay 1 metre away from patient
- handwashing, and cough and sneeze etiquette
- if the patient is in your home, divide the home into different zones for those who are ill and not-ill

---

- when less than 1 metre away from patient, use a mask
- handwashing, cough and sneeze etiquette, and consider gloves if physically caring for her and exposed to her bodily fluids.
- you can still use the zone approach, and be especially vigilant about handwashing when you move from the ill to the not-ill zone

---

- same precautions as for moderate influenza
- if you have just encountered this person, especially outside your own home, consider simply keeping your distance and calling an ambulance if he has very severe symptoms

simply by using the telephone, your best option may be to keep your distance, pick up the phone, and make sure that professional help arrives. Doing this poses no risk to you. If, on the other hand, it is difficult to get medical care because the system is overwhelmed, and you might be able to help a person in this situation by doing the same things you would do for a person with moderate influenza, you will have to decide whether to take this risk.

Only you can decide what risks you will take. Some of the specific information that you may want to consider if you are deciding whether to help someone in a physical way will not be available until a pandemic starts. Here are some of the things to think about, which we should know more about once Phase 6 is under way.

Case Fatality Rate

Of the people who contract influenza, the percentage who die is called the case fatality rate. This number will probably be fairly small. This number may also change over the course of the pandemic. Ask yourself if you can tolerate this risk.

Case Fatality Rates in Specific Age Groups

Most influenza pandemics cause different percentages of people to die in different age groups. If you are in an age group in which very few people die, your risk is different than if you are in an age group where relatively more people die. In all known pandemics, the majority of people in all age groups who have contracted influenza have lived, but there have been differing percentages for differing groups. The actual numbers can't be known until the pandemic starts.

Relative Immunity

Once you've had the pandemic strain of influenza, you probably develop immunity and become much less likely to get it again. If this phenomenon is confirmed during a pandemic, and you have already suffered from and recovered from influenza, it may be a less risky proposition to participate in the physical care of others. On the other hand, because testing will probably not be universally available, you may have to decide whether you've had it based simply upon the kind of illness you had. Some people may be exposed to the virus and have very minimal or mild symptoms, and yet develop immunity to it.

Your Other Medical Issues

If you have other medical problems, especially with your heart or lungs, this increases your chances of developing complications of influenza if you contract this infection.

Is the Medical Care System Working?

Here is a dilemma. If medical care systems are working well during a pandemic, it may be less imperative that you help someone, although your help is likely to be valuable in any scenario. If medical care systems are not working well, you and other lay people may be someone's only source of assistance. Of course, if medical care systems are working well, you may have more confidence that if you become ill, you will actually get good medical attention. If they are not working well, then you may feel unsure of this—which may result in your being less inclined to increase your own personal risk of contracting influenza by delivering care to your neighbour. Mind you, if people don't help one another when they have mild or moderate cases of influenza, it is more likely that medical care systems will be overwhelmed and unable to cope.

It's hard to give you a standard measure of whether medical care systems are working well. During a pandemic, we can predict that there will be lots of positive as well as negative press about health care. The presence of some negative press about health care won't mean that the system isn't functioning, it will just mean that the press is doing what it always does—reporting on news, both good and bad. You'll have to stay abreast of current news and make a judgment call.

ASSESSING AND MONITORING AN ILL PERSON

Vital signs and their trends are signposts to help you understand an ongoing illness in a person. However, don't be obsessed by them. They don't show the whole picture or predict the future. We discuss below some simple kinds of observations that you can make, to help you get a sense of how sick someone is.

Consider taking a first aid course, to learn how to take vital signs and how to assess someone's state of illness. It's worth getting some instruction, because it is often more difficult to determine vital signs in a person who is sick, and especially difficult to do so in a child. A pulse may be weak and faint, and you may be frightened and anxious while trying to find it.

Temperature

Fever itself is not dangerous to a person's health. It is a signpost that there is an infection in the body, which is the important issue. Fever doesn't tell you what the infection is. A person who has a cough, sore muscles, and other symptoms of influenza while a worldwide influenza pandemic happens to be under way probably has influenza. During Phase 6 of a pandemic, such a person should be considered to have it unless a professional medical opinion subsequently diagnoses it as something else. Mind you, even during an influenza pandemic, people will get colds, bladder infections, appendicitis, and other things that cause fever. Just to make it more complicated, influenza can occasionally arrive without a fever, particularly in the elderly.

The main reason to treat a fever with "comfort" medications like acetaminophen (Tylenol) and ibuprofen (Advil, Motrin) is to help the person feel comfortable. A person who feels comfortable may be more able to do important things like drinking lots of fluids.

To take a temperature, you need a thermometer. Many people think that they can tell whether a person has a fever simply by placing a hand on the person's forehead. You can't tell. Equally important, you won't be able to communicate this assessment to anyone if you are trying to get professional advice, either on the phone or in person. "She feels very hot" means very little. Generally, 38°C is a fever, although slightly different numbers apply to different methods of measurement.

A number of thermometers are available. They're all fine. Just find one that you are comfortable using. If you have to share thermometers between people, make sure you wash them in soap and water between uses. Place the end of the glass thermometer under the tongue, and wait a few minutes for the little red line to stop moving. If you put a thermometer under the tongue or under the armpit, add 0.5°C. The ear thermometers are handy, but you're supposed to change the little cover piece each time, which is a pain if you run out of them.

Hydration Status: Urine Output and Heart Rate

Thirst is a very powerful impulse. Most people who are dehydrated feel thirsty, although sometimes if they are sick they feel that they cannot tolerate fluids. Decreased urination and an elevated heart rate should make you wonder if dehydration is a possibility. A dry tongue and dry mouth are clues to dehydration. Sunken eyes, greyish or flushed skin, and decreased skin firmness (doctors call it turgor) happen pretty late. If you see this, a person is probably significantly dehydrated already. Young children, particularly infants, tend to be at higher risk of more rapid dehydration.

The amount of urine that a person produces is an excellent indicator of whether he is getting enough fluid. Over the course of a day, a healthy person should produce 1 millilitre of urine per kilogram of body weight per hour. So an average well-hydrated 70-kilogram person should produce 1.68 litres of urine in a 24-hour period. This is not an especially convenient piece of knowledge, because if you want to know the numbers, you need to collect and measure urine. A person who is urinating less may not be getting enough fluids. Urine that is darker than usual may also suggest some dehydration. A reasonable approximate measure is simply whether a person is urinating as often as usual, and whether he feels that he is producing roughly as much urine as usual.

To assess heart rate, feel for a pulse. In adults and children, an easy place to feel a pulse is the wrist. In infants, feel for the pulse in the groin. If you're not sure where to feel, ask your doctor next time you go in. Heart rate is expressed as beats per minute and should be measured when a person is calm and has been at rest for five minutes. The numbers don't mean the same thing if the person has just run up a flight of stairs. The upper limit of normal for adults is 100. For children, the limits change with age. Fever can increase heart rate. When the resting heart rate is above normal, or the trend is that the resting heart rate is rising above an individual person's usual rate, think about dehydration. In general, when a person does not have enough fluid in her body, her heart rate increases. However, other things can also increase heart rate, and some people who are dehydrated do not have an elevated heart rate. This is more of a clue than an absolute rule, but it's a reasonable clue to watch for.

Rate of Breathing and Effort of Breathing

If someone is consistently breathing faster than normal, has an increased effort of breathing, or has shortness of breath, consider the possibility of pneumonia or another lung complication of influenza. A person with a pre-existing lung condition is more likely to develop such a complication with influenza. These observations should guide your level of concern but not replace a professional assessment.

To measure the rate of breathing, observe a person's chest rising and falling. Count how many cycles he breathes in and out over a full minute to get an accurate measurement. Watch quietly when he doesn't know you are doing it. People often can't help altering their rate of breathing if they know that someone is counting. A normal adult at rest should have a breathing rate between 14 and 20. The normal rate for children will change according to age.

Assessing the effort of breathing is an art, requiring considerable training and experience to make a full assessment. However, here are a few tips. When a person breathes with normal effort, his chest muscles don't visibly move very much, if at all. With additional breathing effort, you may see the muscles between the ribs work, or accentuated movement of the whole chest. You can tell only if his shirt is off. Judging whether chest movement is abnormal or not requires a clear idea of what looks normal. Next time you are at your local pool, check out your fellow swimmers. This will give you some idea of the way that breathing normally appears. When a healthy person is breathing normally, he can do so comfortably in any position. If someone cannot recline but must sit up straight in order to breathe, this is worrisome. His body is trying to maximize the effectiveness of the breathing muscles just to get enough air, and this tells you there is a significant increase in the effort of breathing.

Also important is simply whether the ill person feels short of breath. Shortness of breath is the feeling that it is difficult to get enough air to feel satisfied. It's not the common feeling of "having difficulty breathing" because of a stuffy nose or congestion. With shortness of breath, a person consciously perceives an increased effort to breathe deeper or faster. If someone cannot speak in full sentences, or cannot speak at all because he is using all of his energy to breathe, this is worrisome. He needs medical attention.

The "Gestalt," or "How the Patient Is Doing"

Be mindful of an overall sense of "how the patient is doing." Is the skin healthy-looking, or is it pale, or dusky? Is a person's posture comfortable and relaxed, or is she slumped over because she doesn't have the energy to sit? Alternatively, is she bolt upright because it is the only way she can breathe? How does she interact? Is she communicative and alert, or is she sleepy and slowed down terribly by fatigue? Are her eyes quick and expressive, or are they slow to move and focus?

Pay attention to your impressions of how well a person is doing in this overall way. Although these things sound obvious, they are both subtle and important. There is great power in this type of assessment, much of which happens in a difficult-to-describe and subconscious way. In fact, among the chief things that distinguish an early medical trainee from a seasoned medical professional are not only factual knowledge but also the ability to form an objective yet intuitive impression from simply looking at a patient, an impression that we call a "gestalt." Integrating these types of observations into a professional medical assessment is a skill that usually takes physicians several years to begin to acquire, and that matures over a medical career. On the one hand, it's obvious. On the other, it's not as easy as it sounds.

That being the case, you should rely on your impressions, but err on the side of caution. If you are caring for someone and you think he looks great, then he probably is doing well. If you are caring for someone and think that he looks more sick than before, don't second-guess yourself. Act upon that impression, and seek professional help.

ADULT VITAL SIGNS

VITAL SIGN	HOW TO MEASURE IT
TEMPERATURE	• use a thermometer • leave it under the tongue or armpit for a few minutes • use ear or "tympanic" thermometers as directed by their included instructions
HEART RATE	• feel the wrist, below the base of the thumb using your index and/or middle finger(s) • count for at least 30 seconds, or for a full minute
RATE OF BREATHING	• watch the chest rise and fall and count that as one breath or cycle • count for a full minute • do it when the person is calm and relaxed and doesn't know you're doing it
EFFORT OF BREATHING	• watch the muscles of the chest, and the effort of breathing • if a person can't speak comfortably, that is bad • practise this on normal people, so that you will know what is abnormal
URINE OUTPUT	• for a person who feels well, simply get a rough idea of whether he is urinating as much as usual • if you want to be exact, measure volume of urine

NORMAL	GOOD TO KNOW
• rule of thumb: a fever is 38°C or greater. In reality, the measurement often depends upon which route is used. Add 0.5°C if using the mouth or armpit. Discuss with a health care provider if unsure.	• fever itself is not dangerous; it simply tells you the body has an infection • treating the fever may help someone feel more comfortable
• should be less than 100 at rest; excitement or exertion may increase it • in an individual person, a persistent change from the usual average is also worth noting	• the practical point for you: high heart rate should make you wonder if the person is dehydrated, although it could be something else • fever can increase heart rate, as can anxiety, stress, exertion, and other factors
• normal is 14 to 20 breaths per minute • in an individual person, a persistent change from the usual average is also worth noting • this value can change a great deal from measurement to measurement, so if you're concerned, do it a few times	• the practical point for you: high breathing rate or increased breathing effort should make you wonder if there is pneumonia or another lung complication of influenza • anxiety, stress, and exertion can also increase the rate or effort of breathing
• very minimal visible use of chest muscles • person is able to speak in full sentences while breathing	• don't forget that people with pre-existing lung problems still have them—they need their regular treatments, and are more vulnerable to lung complications of influenza • children breathe faster, even when healthy
• if you are measuring, normal should be 1 cc of urine per kilogram of body weight per hour • in a 70-kilogram adult, this works out to about 1.7 L per day • colour gives you a rough idea—darker implies that urine is more concentrated, and that there is less fluid in body	• decreased urine output and dark urine should make you wonder if the person is dehydrated

Note: This table refers to adults. For children, the normal parameters can change with age. In caring for a child, be in close communication with a health care provider if you need advice, trust your instincts, and err on the side of caution in seeking help.

205

Putting Your Observations in Perspective

Don't obsess about the vital signs and numbers or measure them every five minutes and then panic if one of them is awry. Check twice a day, unless there's a particular reason to do them more often. Keep track of them in a notebook so that you can see trends and changes. Records are useful to help you organize your care of the person, and not an end in themselves. If you're making spreadsheets of vital signs, you're taking it too far.

Although we have given you the standard vital sign numbers used every day by medical professionals, there is ongoing scientific discussion about the predictive value and clinical meaning of these numbers in specific situations. We say this not to discount vital signs, but just to underscore the concept that although we use these numbers as an integral component of assessment in professional health care, they are still signposts that must be viewed in a broader perspective.

Big changes are important. Don't obsess about small ones. For instance, if a person's heart rate is consistently 140 at rest, that's quite fast. Be concerned. If someone else's creeps up to 110 on the occasional measurement but the average is perfectly within the range of normal, don't flip out. Context is important. If you are concerned about someone's vital signs being a little bit off, but she is talking and laughing while eating pizza, you can probably be less concerned. On the other hand, if all of the measurable vital signs are perfect, but the person in question doesn't respond when you shake him vigorously, and his skin is discoloured and mottled, that's not good.

SOME GENERAL TREATMENTS TO HELP
SOMEONE WITH INFLUENZA
Oral Rehydration Solution

Dehydration can make it difficult for a person to recover from illness, and helping someone maintain hydration may be the most important thing you can do. A person who is eating a good, varied diet should drink plenty of whatever fluids she likes. Almost any fluid is fine. The less a person is eating and drinking, or the more she is vomiting or having diarrhea, the more useful it may be for her to drink a specific oral rehydration solution. Rehydration solutions with a specific mix of sugars and electrolytes are available as premade liquids such as Gastrolyte and Pedialyte and also as powders that can be mixed with specified amounts of water.

Sports drinks are not as ideal, because they may contain too much sugar and not enough electrolytes. However, most of the "ideal" rehydration solutions taste saltier than most drinks. Some people don't like them. If a sick person won't drink them, it is better for him to take a "non-ideal" fluid that he likes than to not drink at all. Both alcoholic and caffeinated drinks will make a person lose fluids by urinating excessively, and neither should be used in an attempt to stay hydrated. Milk may irritate the stomach, but there's nothing particularly wrong with it.

ORAL REHYDRATION SOLUTION

INGREDIENTS	OPTIONAL THINGS YOU CAN ADD	GOOD TO KNOW
• 1 L clean water • 40 mL of sugar or honey • 5 mL of salt	• orange or lemon juice: add some for taste, and for potassium • banana, tomato, plantain, or papaya: blend some in for taste, and for potassium • flavour: if it makes it more appealing, flavour with mint, citrus, or vanilla extract	• too sweet is not a dangerous problem, although it may actually worsen diarrhea • too salty can cause dangerous imbalances in the blood, so err on the side of less salty—it shouldn't taste saltier than tears • most adults need a minimum of 2 to 3 litres per day, but many sick people will need more— don't be afraid of giving too much, and if necessary, do it in small amounts such as a few sips every couple of minutes • persons with diarrhea should drink a minimum of one glass per loose bowel movement • anyone should be drinking enough to produce a normal amount of urine

• Make a new batch fresh every day.
• We cannot overemphasize the importance of clean water. Do everything possible to ensure that the water is clean. In developed countries, the safety of the water system is very likely to be preserved during a pandemic.
• Pre-made packets of oral rehydration powder are available and more accurate. You simply add the powder to a volume of clean water. We provide this recipe because it is a standard, well-accepted recipe that is easy to prepare.

"Comfort" medications

Use these to provide comfort and facilitate hydration. When people feel feverish or otherwise sick, they often don't take fluids very well. Fever or nausea are not dangerous in themselves, but the reason to treat them is to help people feel more comfortable and to keep them hydrated. (Antiviral medications will be discussed in a separate chapter.)

Used in its recommended doses, acetaminophen is quite safe for prolonged and ongoing use. Ibuprofen works well in treating fever, but be aware that it can irritate the stomach. Prolonged use can be complicated by bleeding of the stomach. Dimenhydrinate (Gravol) can be used to treat nausea, and this may assist greatly in helping someone to stay hydrated.

COMFORT MEDICATIONS

PROBLEM	COMFORT MEASURE	HOW TO USE IT IN ADULTS	HOW TO USE IT IN CHILDREN
FEVER, PAIN	Acetaminophen (brand names: Tylenol, Tempra)	Up to 1,000 mg every four hours, maximum of 4,000 mg per day	10 to 15 mg per kg of child's weight, every four hours as needed
	Ibuprofen (brand names: Advil, Motrin)	Up to 200 to 400 mg every six hours, maximum of 2,400 mg per day	4 to 10 mg per kg of child's weight, every six to eight hours as needed, maximum of 50 mg per kg per day
NAUSEA	Dimenhydrinate (brand name: Gravol)	Up to 50 to 100 mg every four hours, maximum of 400 mg per day	consult product literature

WHEN TO ASK A PROFESSIONAL BEFORE USING

GOOD TO KNOW

WHEN TO ASK A PROFESSIONAL BEFORE USING	GOOD TO KNOW
• alcoholism • hepatitis • liver disease • taking other drugs that place demands upon the liver	• Acetaminophen and ibuprofen can be safely used together at each of their maximum doses, for more fever control and pain relief. • You can give them at alternating times, or together, whichever works best. • These give relief for only a few hours, so don't be surprised when the fever and pain come back.
• asthma that is sensitive to ASA/NSAID • stomach ulcer or bleeding in the digestive tract • third-trimester of pregnancy	
• for a child less than two years old • note: this medication is generally not used in children less than one year old	• This drug will also make people drowsy.

CHAPTER 10

THE IMPORTANCE OF ANIMAL HEALTH TO HUMAN HEALTH

THIS CHAPTER IN ONE PAGE . . .

- Domestic poultry can become infected with highly pathogenic influenza strains, such as H5N1, which can infect humans and potentially contribute to starting a pandemic.
- Poorer countries often use high-risk agricultural practices, where animals and humans as well as wild and domestic birds share a common space and interact closely. This gives the influenza virus opportunity to spread among different species of birds and to become adapted to infecting humans. Changing these practices can be culturally and economically difficult for subsistence farmers.
- Culling domestic bird flocks to control outbreaks of infection is sometimes necessary but can be damaging to farmers and the industry.
- Vaccination of domestic birds is controversial but can help control H5N1 infections in farms.
- Bird-to-human transmission of H5N1 occurs through close contact with the secretions and excretions of sick birds.
- Birders and hunters should use caution if they handle birds in the wild.
- The trade of birds, especially that of the contraband market, may also play a role in the spread of influenza strains like H5N1.
- Other animals, including mammals, can be affected by H5N1.
- Handling and cooking chicken from the supermarket is safe, and you should always take care to wash your hands and utensils thoroughly.

"Birds carrying the virus along the West African—Atlantic flyway will move into the area of Greenland and Northern Canada and then, probably towards the latter parts of this year, move down into the American continent."
—David Nabarro, WHO and Senior UN System Coordinator for Avian and Human Influenza, March 9, 2006[1]

DOMESTIC POULTRY: THE CRUCIAL LINK FOR AVIAN INFLUENZA IN HUMANS

At the time of writing, the H5N1 virus has caused massive outbreaks in Asian bird flocks and has spread to over 50 countries in the Middle East, Africa, and Europe, causing dramatic outbreaks in birds in some places and sporadic human illnesses. Some expect that H5N1 will soon reach North America, and this may have happened by the time you read this. However, not all experts agree upon the role of migratory birds in spreading the virus. The role of domestic poultry flocks is better understood and is a key link between strains of avian influenza, including H5N1, and human beings. Domestic chickens, ducks, and other birds pass it to humans. These principles are not unique to H5N1, as strains of other avian influenzas are constantly circulating in birds.

People who live and work with domestic birds need to use farming and handling practices that minimize the chance that infections can be transmitted between domestic and wild fowl, and that such viruses might jump from birds to humans. People who raise or interact with birds must know how to detect illness that may represent worrisome strains of influenza. Each individual human infection is an opportunity for a strain of influenza to adapt more to humans. When a worrisome strain of influenza, such as H5N1, enters domestic poultry flocks, sick birds are culled. Birds that are not ill but are at risk of developing disease may be culled or immunized. People who are in contact with birds need to be monitored for illnesses that may represent an infection with a concerning strain of influenza.

The H5N1 strain of influenza is currently spreading throughout the world's wild and domestic bird populations, and its range is expanding. Whether wild birds serve to spread the H5N1 strain of influenza over large distances is the subject of controversy. Although at first glance it seems plausible that migrating birds could play this role, the pattern and timing of several domestic bird flu outbreaks have not corresponded with periods of major wild bird migrations or their migratory routes. Certainly, the deaths of wild birds have been associated with outbreaks of H5N1 in poultry, but it is not clear whether the wild birds were the source of the virus, or whether they themselves were victims and were infected through interaction with domestic poultry, which in turn may have acquired the virus through some other route. However wild birds are infected, they may still play a role in spreading the infection, even if only among domestic birds within a local area. The science is still young. Before the most recent H5N1 outbreak, not enough surveillance of wild birds occurred to answer these questions. Scientists are now setting up surveillance systems worldwide to track H5N1 in migrating birds.

It is not recommended that wild birds be culled or otherwise interfered with for the purpose of controlling the spread of H5N1 influenza, or any other strain of influenza. The role of these birds in spreading viruses across large geographical distances is unclear. A complete cull of a wild bird population would be impossible, and the ecological consequences of any such attempt are unknown and potentially disastrous. In addition to potentially major ecological disruption, there could be human health consequences that we cannot predict.

The global trade of birds, legal and illegal, either as exotic pets or for use in activities such as cockfighting, may play a role in the global spread of H5N1. Some experts feel that this trade may actually pose a more important and greater risk of introducing H5N1 to North America than the possible importation of the virus by migratory birds. Dr. Lonnie King of the Centers for Disease Control estimates that the annual global trade in exotic animals includes 4 million birds, 640,000 reptiles, and 140,000 primates a year.[2] There is a parallel contraband trade in these exotic animals with a value of U.S. $4 billion to $6 billion per year, which is second in value only to the global illegal drug trade.[2] If the bird trade brings the virus here, it would not be the first time a serious infection has arrived in North America via trade in animals. In 2003, monkey pox arrived in the United States through the importation of Gambian giant rats from Ghana, West Africa, via a Texas animal distributor. Those rats then infected prairie dogs that made their way to an Illinois dealer, who sold them to families as pets. Thirty-five people were then infected with monkey pox by the prairie dogs.[3]

If migratory birds eventually do play a role in bringing H5N1 to North America, some experts, such as Dr. Leslie Dierauf, a wildlife veterinarian at the United States National Wildlife Health Center, believe that it will probably occur through the Alaska-Bering Strait, instead of the Atlantic Ocean flyway.[4] In the spring, migratory birds from North America move north to their summer feeding grounds.[5] There they can interact with migratory birds from Asia. For example, there is a species of loon that flies from Alaska across the Bering Strait to northern Japan in the winter and returns to Alaska in the summer. When the North American birds move south in August and September, there is a possibility that they may bring with them viral strains acquired from their Asian counterparts. The summer of 2006 saw surveillance of wild birds for H5N1 both on the east coast of North America and in Alaska by the Canadian Wildlife Services and the U.S. Geological Survey. Telephone hotlines to report sightings of dead birds exist in England and may be established in North America this year for that purpose. The approach is similar to that introduced in previous summers in some parts of Canada for the purpose of West Nile virus control; public health hotlines to report sightings of dead crows were set up to ensure that dead birds could be collected and tested.

Thai Eagles in Brussels[6]

On October 18, 2005, H5N1 made its first known appearance in Europe, when a Thai man was stopped at Zaventem Airport, in Brussels, for a random drug check. Within his hand luggage, packed into plastic tubes, customs officers found two small, crested hawk eagles. These eagles are an endangered species, and the man had no permits for their transport or trade. In addition, the European Union had banned the importation of all birds from countries affected by H5N1.

The eagles, in poor physical condition and barely alive, had to be sacrificed. Two days later, Belgian authorities ordered tests for strains of avian influenza and discovered that the deceased birds had been infected by the H5N1 virus. A country-wide manhunt was launched for the smuggler, who had not been detained because Belgian law does not provide for the detention of smugglers. The smuggler subsequently turned himself in at an Antwerp hospital, and as a precaution, some 700 birds, mainly canaries that were in the animal quarantine area of the Zaventem airport, were sacrificed. Human contacts of the birds were treated with Tamiflu.

The H5N1 strain of influenza has since come to affect several European countries. The current outbreaks are not linked to the Brussels incident. Since much bird smuggling activity goes undetected, the degree to which some bird owners may be at increased risk of being exposed to H5N1 is unknown. The exact mechanism by which H5N1 spreads over large geographic distances is still a subject of scientific inquiry. To be safe, if you decide to buy a pet bird, ensure it has appropriate importation and health certificates.

HIGH-RISK BIRD AGRICULTURE

One of the chief reasons that human cases of H5N1 have occurred mostly in Asia is the high density of people living in Asia who raise birds using high-risk methods. Households in poorer countries raise birds and pigs in their backyards, where children play, and some allow the animals to enter the human home. Wild birds interact with free-range domestic birds. Children play with birds and may contract infections from them. In some places, fighting cocks are prized household assets that are allowed to roam freely in homes. Sick birds are sometimes consumed by the household, so a family may handle virus-contaminated raw meat. Live birds are sold and slaughtered in crowded "wet" markets, where thousands of birds of different species are sold, and where there is ample opportunity for infections to spread between birds. Unsold birds are often returned to the village where they came from, so that a bird that has acquired an infection at market but not been sold can take the virus home. Although they are rare, live bird markets do exist in North America.

Asia is certainly not the only part of the world where poultry is raised in high-risk ways. Africa, the Middle East, and South America all have large populations of people who raise birds in small households and farms using practices similar to those in Asia. These provide the setting for a new influenza strain to make the jump from domestic poultry to humans.

To date, there has been no animal-to-human transmission of H5N1 within a fully industrialized poultry production system using an industry-accepted level of biosecurity measures. Certainly, commercial farms have experienced outbreaks among their poultry, but to date it hasn't jumped to humans in this setting. This doesn't mean that industrial systems are foolproof, or that animal-to-human transmission couldn't happen in such a setting. In 2004, there was an outbreak of a different strain (not H5N1) of avian influenza in poultry in the Fraser Valley region of British Columbia that resulted in two human infections and the eventual culling of 15 million birds.

Commercial poultry systems are certainly vulnerable to outbreaks among their flocks because huge numbers of birds are often crowded into very limited spaces, and the genetic similarity of many of the birds in a large industrial poultry farm may make all these birds similarly susceptible to an infection. The appearance of H5N1 in a commercial bird farm is often not subtle: it can cause the majority of birds in a crowded flock to die suddenly. Nonetheless, it is important for bird farmers to be vigilant for quieter appearances of this virus.

The rarity of animal-to-human transmission of H5N1 and other avian influenza strains in industrial farms in richer countries does demonstrate the principle that there are identifiable high-risk farming practices that increase the risk of a potentially dangerous influenza strain making the jump to people. These high-risk practices need to be identified and changed.

Dr. Lee's Perspective
Chickens in Rural Asia

As a child growing up in Malaysia, I chased chickens in and out of my grandmother's house on sweltering afternoons, sometimes because they were to be the meal of the day but mostly just for fun. Sometimes my grandmother would point out a chicken that she wanted in the pot and send us after it. We might chase it through the yard, into the house, and back into the yard before being able to corner it and bring it, squawking and struggling, to the chopping block. Cockfights were commonplace, where crowds would press around a pair of roosters fighting for their male pride as well as for their masters. For someone who owned a strong, nasty fighting cock, the bird was often a prime source of cash income and a prized possession, and an owner would demonstrate this to others by giving the rooster a kiss on the beak after a victory.

I often accompanied my grandmother on meat and vegetable shopping to a "wet market" near her home. Hundreds of ducks and chickens clucked in an open air market, the ground constantly wet with water used to clear away bird feces and blood from slaughtering. My grandmother would handle and inspect live birds to choose the "fattest" one, which represented the best value. As I write this, I am preparing to travel to H5N1-affected areas in Southeast Asia to visit my family. As always, I expect that my grandmother would like me to accompany her to the market.

CHANGING FARMING PRACTICES

Making changes to farming practices requires the education of farmers at a relevant local and individual level. The reasons to change traditional practices may not immediately be clear to an individual farmer. The methods that small farmers use to raise birds are often part of a precarious way of earning a living. These birds are an often important source of dietary protein and cash income, and changing farming practices may generate more work for farmers and reduce their incomes. Many subsistence farmers in a poor country do not have access to the worldwide media or the perspective that the reader of this book is more likely to have. Since human cases of H5N1 are still quite rare within any small local area, it may be difficult for farmers to accept the culling of their flocks of chickens, even if diseased, or the implementation of a new farming practice that might disrupt their fragile household economy. Any change in such practices requires education at a local level that is relevant and that provides viable alternative ways to raise animals.

Any kind of intervention must also compensate people for their losses. If a country can't pay for the birds that must be destroyed, or can't pay for upgrading agricultural practices, the measures won't work. When we hear about culls, we must understand that in a poor country, these measures disrupt both a family's food supply and its cash flow. As of March 2006, the WHO estimated that the culling of poultry in Asia and other places has affected over 300 million subsistence farmers with an estimated economic impact of over US$10 billion, much of this borne directly by poor rural farmers.[2]

What can we do in rich countries? First, we should realize that although most of our farming practices are distinctly lower in risk, we are not exempt from concern. A new strain of influenza could still enter our poultry farming system, and the species jump from animal to human could still happen in our commercial farms. Remember that one strong contender for the genesis of the 1918–19 influenza was rural Kansas, although it was a poorer and more subsistence-economy-based state in that time. Even today, the richest countries have people who raise poultry in their households, as a hobby or for personal consumption. At present, North America has not seen H5N1 in domesticated poultry. We must ensure that our own farming practices limit the interaction between wild birds and farm birds by ensuring that the farm birds are in enclosed quarters, that birds and their human handlers are closely monitored for disease, that timely testing is done, and that contact between humans and birds takes place in a controlled and clean manner. Free-range birds may need to be kept indoors to eliminate the possibility of interaction with wild birds. Even with the highest standard of precautions and interventions, H5N1 or other avian influenzas may enter domestic poultry flocks. Despite the well-developed animal health infrastructure in France, H5N1 was found in that country in February 2006.

Human handlers of birds must be well educated about the issue of farming practices and influenza, and must pay particular attention during slaughtering, when the birds' bodily fluids and feces are potentially in close contact with them. The human handlers of birds should all receive the annual influenza vaccine, certainly in rich countries and ideally also in poor ones. One possible mechanism for the eruption of a pandemic is a genetic reassortment between an influenza strain that resides in birds and another such as seasonal influenza strain that resides and spreads easily among humans. Some argue that immunizing bird handlers reduces the probability that one individual may be co-infected with two strains of influenza, whose combination could produce a virus of pandemic potential. In rich countries, this may be easier to achieve because we have fewer people who are in contact with birds as a proportion of our population and we can afford to pay for the vaccination of such numbers of people.

In affluent countries, we should support attempts at controlling potentially dangerous strains of avian influenza in the agricultural economies of poor countries, both financially and scientifically. Some feel that affluent countries have not done enough to support agricultural control measures in poorer countries. On March 6, 2006, the French daily *Libération* reported the comments of the head of the Food and Agriculture Organization of the UN, Jacques Diouf, upon the appearance of H5N1 in western Europe: "Governments have sinned by failing to look ahead and have a sense of solidarity . . . Developed countries thought that this was going on in Asia, that it was far away and that we were exaggerating the risks of the epidemic."[7]

Faraway poultry farming issues are our poultry farming issues, and distant agricultural control measures have a direct link to our worldwide risk of pandemic influenza. The rural Thai chicken farmer who develops a fever and a cough is a mere motorcycle ride away from the capital, Bangkok, where he visits with his cousin who is a porter at a five-star hotel full of vacationing Westerners.

The Successful but Expensive Control of H5N1 in Hong Kong

Hong Kong experienced H5N1 outbreaks in domestic poultry in 1997, 2001, and 2002. The 1997 outbreak caused 18 human cases with 6 deaths; it was followed by the culling of all 1.5 million commercial poultry in the country in 3 days and the closure of poultry markets for months. Since then, drastic changes in farming and marketing practices have been used to control H5N1. Despite widespread H5N1 outbreaks ravaging neighbouring countries, such as Vietnam, Cambodia, and Thailand, since 2003, cases of H5N1 have not been found in Hong Kong domestic poultry.

What measures are currently being taken?

• "Birdproofing" of farms: no interaction between wild and domestic birds; prohibition of bird movement between farms.

• Equipment: plastic and metal bird cages only (no wood) that are easily disinfected daily; protective equipment for farmers.

• Testing for infection: dead birds tested; random testing of live birds from farms and markets; testing of cages from farms and markets.

• Vaccination: H5 vaccination and testing of vaccinated flocks for adequate antibodies.

• Prohibition of "backyard" poultry: hefty fine for non-compliance.

• Limited importation of birds into Hong Kong: 20,000 per day, health certificates required.

• Market rest days twice a month: all commercial poultry removed from markets for 18 hours to "break the infection cycle" and to allow thorough cleaning and disinfection of the markets.

• Centralization of slaughter sites: fewer potentially H5N1-contaminated sites and more consistent hygienic slaughter practices.

• Reducing the poultry population: the goal is to have only 2 million birds.

What is the cost?

• HK$270 million (C$40 million) of compensation was given to poultry farmers between 1997 and 2004.

• HK$600 million (C$90 million) is being offered to help traders who opt for voluntary exit from the trade and cease operation permanently.

References:

Presentation from T. Ellis, Murdoch University, Australia—Risk Management for Poultry Production and Marketing in a H5N1 Endemic Region, at the 2006 International Conference on Emerging Infectious Diseases held in Atlanta, Georgia.

Hong Kong Special Administrative Region press release on March 15, 2006, accessed on March 22, 2006, at http://www.info.gov.hk/gia/general/200603/15/P2006031 50203.htm

VACCINATION

Another way to limit the spread of H5N1 in birds is to vaccinate them. The advantage of vaccination is that it can prevent disease and potentially save the poultry industry of a country from collapse, in the event of a widespread outbreak that would otherwise trigger widespread culling as the only control option.[8] It is easier for farmers to cooperate when their flocks are not faced with destruction. Vaccination decreases the viral load and the likelihood of transmission among birds and, by extension, the likelihood of transmission to humans and the possibility of the emergence of a pandemic strain. It will probably not, however, be able to eradicate H5N1.

An argument against vaccination has to do with the phenomenon of asymptomatic transmission.[8] Vaccination may not completely prevent virus from infecting a flock, or prevent the birds from shedding virus. Therefore, a novel strain of influenza might enter a poultry flock asymptomatically—without visible signs of illness or deaths. This occurred with a different strain of influenza for which a vaccine was administered to poultry in Mexico, Central America, and Asia. Asymptomatic transmission among birds might pose a greater risk to humans since there would not be the same degree of warning in the form of obvious bird disease.

Just as important as the vaccination is the ability to differentiate between infected and vaccinated birds, and therefore good surveillance is necessary to accompany a vaccination program. Italy has been vaccinating a proportion of its poultry since 1999, but it was initially shut out of the export market because of skepticism about vaccination. Also, vaccination does not help farmers to improve isolation, disease control, or biosecurity measures.

There is no universal agreement on the question of whether vaccination is the right or wrong thing to do, but with the current worldwide H5N1 outbreaks in poultry, many countries are choosing this option. Early in 2006, China announced its intention to immunize all of its 7 billion chickens. Some observers criticized this move, partly because of fears that suboptimal vaccines might be sold and used in China. France, Holland, and Russia have also decided to vaccinate their poultry flocks following the arrival of H5N1 there. Many contend that culling is a better, more definitive option, although even culling strategies have not universally stopped the spread of H5N1 in affected countries.

EATING CHICKEN

If you like to eat chicken or poultry, you can continue. The way that people probably contract influenza from sick poultry is from the handling and preparation of the bird before it is cooked. Tigers and cats have contracted H5N1 from eating raw dead birds. Adequate cooking of poultry destroys the influenza virus. If you do want to take any extra precautions regarding birds, be very careful in the cleaning and preparation of poultry. It is not recommended that diseased birds be sold or eaten, and if you know that your pet turkey is sick, it would not be advisable to pluck and dress it for a meal. Meanwhile, the truth is that you wouldn't get influenza from eating the turkey even if it did have influenza, but you may pick it up if you're stuffing the bird before it's cooked and you touch your eyes, nose, or mouth with your contaminated hands.

PETS AND OTHER ANIMALS

If H5N1 becomes prevalent in the wild birds where you live, it may be prudent to keep your cats indoors and to keep your dogs on leashes. Domestic cats have been seen to contract H5N1 and die from it, presumably from eating infected birds. Cats have been found to be infected in Asia since 2003. At the end of February 2006, a domestic cat was killed by H5N1 on the island of Ruegen, Germany. Cats may be able to transmit H5N1 to one another, although this has never been clearly observed. It is unlikely that domestic cats play a role in the usual transmission life cycle of H5N1. It is theoretically possible that cats could transmit this infection to humans. But since the risk of cats contracting H5N1 is quite low, the risk to their human companions is judged to be correspondingly low. In 2005, studies by the National Institute of Animal Health in Bangkok showed that dogs are also able to contract the H5N1 virus. At the time of this writing, there is less clear information regarding the potential for H5N1 to cause illness in dogs. A suggestion of avian influenza in a deceased dog in Azerbaijan has been made. If dogs can be affected by H5N1, there is at least a theoretical possibility that they may be able to pass it to their owners. The risk to dogs is low and at present is poorly understood, and the risk to their human owners is felt to be correspondingly low.

FAO Recommendations

These are the Food and Agriculture Organization of the United Nations recommendations in areas where highly pathogenic H5N1 has been diagnosed or is suspected in poultry or wild birds.[9]

- Report to the local veterinary authority any evidence of significant bird mortality, both wild and domestic.
- Be especially vigilant for any dead or sick cats and report such findings to the local vet.
- Make sure contact between cats and wild birds or poultry (or their feces) is avoided and/or keep cats inside.
- If cats bring a sick or dead bird inside the house, put on plastic gloves and dispose of the bird in a plastic bag for collection by local veterinary animal handlers.
- Keep stray cats outside the house and avoid contact with them.
- If cats show breathing problems or nasal discharge, a veterinarian should be consulted.
- Do not touch or handle any sick-looking or dead cat (or other animal), and report it to the authorities.
- Wash hands with water and soap regularly and especially after handling animals and cleaning their

litter boxes or coming in contact with feces or saliva.

- Dogs can be taken outside the premises only if kept under restraint.
- Do not feed any water birds.
- Disinfect (e.g., with bleach 2–3%) cages or other hardware with which sick animals have been transported or been in contact.
- Wash animal blankets with soap or any other commercial detergent.

Some have pointed to the black market trade in exotic pets and birds as a potential avenue for the spread of H5N1 influenza. Such birds and animals do not undergo the same animal health inspections as legal birds upon importation, and you would be well advised to avoid them. Fatal outbreaks of H5N1 in Thai zoo tigers occurred in 2003 and 2004. The tigers were probably initially exposed to H5N1 through their diet of raw chickens, but it was also demonstrated that the tigers were probably able to pass the infection from tiger to tiger. Tigers, whose numbers in captivity in the U.S. are believed to rival the rest of the world's wild tiger population, are but one of the many unusual animals sometimes kept as exotic pets. There has been no demonstrated spread of H5N1 from tigers to humans, but you should never get very close to tigers anyway.

A common bird that we encounter in North America is the pigeon, a creature that is relatively innocuous. We must note that domestic pigeons have been implicated in the transmission of H5N1 to humans who subsequently died of H5N1 infection in Iraq. In birds, influenza typically affects the digestive tract. If you are in a place where H5N1 is present in birds, it would be prudent to avoid bird droppings and close contact with local bird species that could potentially be infected by H5N1. However, there is no need to overdo it by being afraid of birds. You should treat them with just as much respect as other wild animals and not get too close to them.

The mammals that at this time are known to be susceptible to H5N1, by way of natural observation or demonstration in a laboratory, are palm civet cats, domestic cats, cynomolgus macaques, stone martens, ferrets, New Zealand white rabbits, leopards, tigers, rats, pigs, and humans.

Hunters and Birders

Some of the 75 known wild bird hosts of H5N1 include ducks, geese, swans, gulls, shorebirds, sparrows, starlings, and pigeons. Hunters shoot, handle, and sometimes consume migratory birds, and the geographical range of H5N1 is continually expanding. In some countries, hunters are recruited as part of surveillance networks to monitor the spread of H5N1. This approach may be a way to engage this group of people and educate them about safe bird handling practices. On the other hand, in affluent countries where this is a sport, some may argue that we should just stop hunting birds.

Why allow this potential venue for exposure, in places where it is a recreational activity? It's difficult to quantify the personal risk from bird hunting, which is low. However, H5N1 may soon have a presence on all continents in wild bird populations. It is clear that handling infected birds presents a threat to the handler, and each human infection is a fresh opportunity for H5N1 to adapt itself better to humans and potentially become a virus of pandemic potential. If a recreational activity creates these potential risks, even to a small degree, perhaps it should be halted. To put this suggestion in context, what we ask of Asia and other poor countries is that they engage in large-scale animal control practices that drastically affect the viability of poor, rural subsistence economies. For us to restrain ourselves from shooting birds for sport is a comparatively minuscule inconvenience.

Bird hunters may consider taking up birdwatching. If you are a birder, you can continue to watch from a distance. In general, wild birds don't give disease to humans because wild birds and humans don't generally have physical contact unless one of them is shot. Birders should remember that avian influenza generally inhabits the digestive tracts of birds, so birders should avoid bird feces and clean themselves carefully if they do come in contact with bird excrement. Certainly, birders should not handle birds found to be ill or dying, without guidance and assistance from knowledgeable wildlife and animal health workers.

CHAPTER 11

THE RACE FOR A PANDEMIC VACCINE

THIS CHAPTER IN ONE PAGE . . .

- A vaccine works by giving the body a chance to learn how to recognize and defend itself against an infectious agent.
- Vaccines have an excellent safety record.
- Vaccines are specific to particular virus strains.
- The development of vaccines is unattractive to many pharmaceutical companies for business reasons.
- Using current technology, it would take at least four to six months following the start of a pandemic to create a new specific vaccine for the pandemic strain of influenza.
- Once a new vaccine is created, production can start, but worldwide capacity is limited.
- New technologies for vaccine development and production are being explored.
- During an influenza pandemic, there may be a fast-track process to put new vaccines quickly into use.
- Vaccine will be distributed according to a defined priority list.
- The decision to embark upon a vaccination campaign may be a difficult judgment, weighing the damage caused by a potential or ongoing pandemic as well as what is known and unknown about a new vaccine.

VACCINE PRIORITY GROUPS IN THE 1957–58 PANDEMIC

"By the end of next year, Canada would have produced some 600,000 doses of vaccine. Distribution is due to start next month. Since there isn't enough for everyone, key personnel and essential services will be the first to be immunized. I have learned by the way that this does not apply to Prime Minister Diefenbaker, members of cabinet, MPs and senators. Because of the upcoming royal visit, however, members of the Governor General's staff will be vaccinated."
—CBC reporter Arthur Blakeley, "The Asian flu arrives in Canada," broadcast, September 29, 1957[1]

WHAT CAN VACCINES DO?

The only intervention that may definitively change the direction of an influenza pandemic once it is under way is a timely, effective vaccine. To achieve this outcome, such a vaccine would have to be quickly developed, produced in large quantities, and delivered rapidly around the world to protect as many people as possible. Vaccination was used as early as 1796, dating back to the inoculation of people against smallpox. Seasonal influenza vaccines have been used since 1945, and routine childhood immunizations, with a very good safety record, serve in many countries to prevent a host of previously devastating childhood illnesses. You would think that this collective experience and knowledge would allow us to almost immediately produce a vaccine for pandemic influenza in response to this threat to human health. However, the scientific difficulties associated with producing a specific and effective vaccine, as well as the business issues related to vaccine development and production, pose obstacles to the timely production of a vaccine against a pandemic strain of influenza. Hopefully, we will successfully implement effective public health measures such as containment measures for individuals and communities during an influenza pandemic. A major reason for implementing these measures is to buy time to develop an effective vaccine.

Thanks to vaccination, smallpox has been eradicated, while in North America, polio, measles, diphtheria, tetanus, and rubella infections are rarely heard of. These illnesses once posed ongoing and significant threats to human health in Canada, and achieving these successes through vaccination took decades of concerted efforts on the part of vaccine makers as well as public health workers.

In some places in the developed world, there is an almost complacent attitude toward vaccinations, and in certain small quarters there is outright hostility and opposition to vaccination. It should be noted that where immunization rates have dropped, rates of disease and death have often increased. In 2000, following a drop in measles immunization rates, Ireland had 1,200 cases of measles and saw the deaths of several children, in comparison with 148 cases in 1999.[2] In 1994, 5,000 deaths from diphtheria occurred in Russia following the suspension of the organized immunization system, whereas the country had previously seen only sporadic and unusual cases of this infection.[2] Within the span of a few weeks in 2005, in a community with low rubella vaccination rates in Oxford County, Ontario, there were almost 300 cases of rubella, which regrettably included pregnant women.[3] Infants born to these infected women are at risk of congenital rubella syndrome, which can cause problems with their eyes, heart, hearing, and neurological and cognitive development.

For most childhood and other preventable illnesses, the actual vaccine is only one component of a vaccination program. Such a program must have the capacity to produce sufficient vaccine, to distribute it widely, and to monitor those who are vaccinated for both the effectiveness and side effects. The 500,000 deaths a year worldwide of children under the age of five due to vaccine-preventable measles infections are an ongoing tragedy, largely attributable to the lack of effective vaccination programs.[4] An influenza pandemic happens only occasionally and then runs its course over a small number of years. One of the challenges of vaccination as a response to an influenza pandemic is that the opportunity within which a vaccine intervention may make a difference is relatively short, and the scope of the enterprise is daunting. An influenza pandemic unfolds in a much briefer period than the usual time needed to develop, produce, and distribute an effective vaccine to a huge number of people.

HOW VACCINES WORK

A vaccine works by giving the body a chance to learn how to recognize an infectious agent. A vaccine is similar in molecular shape and appearance to the infectious agent it protects against. When a vaccine is introduced into a human body, the body's immune system can practise defending itself against the infectious agent with that shape, without having to fend off an actual infection. This means that when this body is exposed to the actual infectious agent, it is much better equipped to fight it effectively. Because infectious agents have a huge variety of specific shapes and appearances, vaccines need to be correspondingly specific. "Attenuated" vaccines contain very weak versions of a live virus. "Inactivated" vaccines contain virus that has been inactivated by heat and chemicals.

VACCINES FOR THE NEXT PANDEMIC

We produce a new seasonal influenza vaccine each year, but with current technology we can produce a specific pandemic vaccine only once the pandemic arrives. Research to develop new, "cross-protective" vaccines has begun.

Every year's seasonal influenza vaccine is a little different from the previous season's. Different strains and subtypes of influenza virus circulate from season to season, undergoing constant change. Months ahead of the actual influenza season, influenza watchers predict the three subtypes that they believe will probably circulate in the next season and ask the vaccine manufacturers to produce a corresponding vaccine. Sometimes these predictions are wrong, and a subtype not found in the vaccine circulates prominently during the next season. This can decrease the effectiveness of the vaccine tremendously. There is no "universal" vaccine that is effective for all seasonal influenza subtypes and for the next pandemic.

Although there are current human cases of H5N1 infection, these strains do not travel easily from human to human and are not pandemic-causing strains. A number of H5N1 vaccine trials are ongoing, using human volunteers. The United States plans to stockpile 20 million doses of an H5N1 vaccine for early use in the event of an H5N1 pandemic. The problem is that the virus we see today must change if it is to become a pandemic-causing virus. To what degree these changes will affect the efficacy of the H5N1 vaccine designed on the basis of the structure of the current H5N1 strain of virus is unknown. If the virus changes significantly enough, a more specific vaccine may have to be formulated once the changes are known. Also, we cannot be certain that H5N1 will cause the next influenza pandemic, although it is certainly the clearest present threat.

Scientists are currently working hard and making progress on producing a vaccine that would be effective for all influenza A virus strains, including the next pandemic strain. This would be called a "cross-protective" vaccine.[5-7] Even if this vaccine were only 50% effective during a pandemic, it would not only prevent millions of infections but would buy time for scientists to characterize the pandemic strain and produce a more specific and effective vaccine. We are probably still years away from having such a cross-protective vaccine.

VACCINE DEVELOPMENT

The development of vaccines is unattractive to many pharmaceutical companies for business reasons. It is an expensive, slow process with uncertain financial returns. During an influenza pandemic, there may be a fast-track process to put new vaccines into use.

It takes many millions of dollars to develop, test, license, produce, and market a new vaccine. A company has no guarantee of any demand for that vaccine. It is easier for a company to assess the market demand for a pill that treats a condition: it can find out how many people have that condition. It is harder to assess market demand for a preventive strategy like vaccination, because this depends upon people or governments deciding that it is worthwhile for people to be protected against an illness. The commercial prospects for a pandemic influenza vaccine are highly unpredictable. The timing of the pandemic and therefore the timing of demand for such a vaccine are unknown. Seasonal influenza vaccine is currently produced in only nine countries, including Canada and the United States. About 70% of all influenza vaccines are produced in Europe.

Since vaccines are "biologic drugs" and injected into people, the safety regulations created by bodies such as Health Canada and the U.S. Food and Drug Administration (FDA) are understandably quite stringent. It is generally easier to develop and license a pill. It is also more profitable to develop medications that a person takes daily, such as a blood pressure or cholesterol treatment, than a vaccine that may be needed only once in someone's life. In order to counter these disincentives, it has been suggested that specific financial and economic incentives be offered to promote new vaccine development. These might include pricing that accounts for research and development costs, guaranteed purchase of unsold supplies, tax incentives, liability protection, and intellectual property considerations.

In the United States, the FDA has "investigational new drug" provisions and the emergency-use authorization of medical products that would allow new vaccines to be used more rapidly during the pandemic, without the prolonged testing and licensing procedures applicable to most new vaccines.[8-9] They would have to be strictly monitored for side effects, and if a high number of serious side effects were observed, such that the risks of the new vaccines were felt to outweigh the benefits, it might be necessary to stop using them.

VACCINE PRODUCTION

Using current technology it will take months following the start of a pandemic to create a new vaccine. From the moment the strain is located, the process of isolating and characterizing the virus, then creating an effective vaccine and testing it to ensure an adequate level of safety and effectiveness, would take at least four to six months. Once a new vaccine is created, production of the vaccine can start. Traditional manufacturing techniques have some limitations and do not allow for rapid increases in production capacity. New methods are being explored.

The manufacture of influenza vaccines is a slow process, based on a venerable technique using fertilized chicken eggs that was developed more than 50 years ago. The eggshell is cracked, and the influenza virus strain is injected into the fluid surrounding the embryo. The egg is resealed, and the embryo becomes infected, allowing the virus to reproduce. The resulting virus is harvested, purified, inactivated so that it does not cause an actual infection, and used to produce the vaccine. Using this method, production of seasonal influenza vaccines requires about one egg per dose. Immunization against a pandemic strain is expected to require two doses per person, one month apart. For the 6.3 billion people on earth, that's 12.6 billion eggs. That's a lot of eggs to get hold of, especially if worldwide outbreaks of avian influenza are decimating domestic chicken flocks. Another potential problem is that the pandemic strain of influenza might kill the eggs during the vaccine manufacturing process. It's also thought that for a pandemic strain of influenza, each person may require a higher dose of vaccine than a typical seasonal influenza dose, so that could require even more eggs.

A number of new vaccine production methods are being developed. Once the pandemic strain is isolated and characterized, vaccinologists need to create a "master" seed virus strain that is not dangerous to humans but will also produce a human immunological response in a vaccine. There are molecular and genetic methods being studied to speed up this process.[10]

Another novel approach is a cell-based method, using giant vats of living cells. It would be much quicker to increase production by using this method and a seed strain than by using individually harvested and purified egg-based vaccines. Yet another method in development called subunit vaccination would entail injecting a fragment of influenza DNA instead of purified virus into a person. The injected DNA would then produce the influenza proteins against which an immune system would mount a response. There would be a shorter production time, because we can produce large quantities of specific DNA sequences using laboratory techniques, without needing to rely upon eggs or other living organisms. These and other experimental methods of vaccine production are probably still years away from becoming a reality, but the science is ongoing. A technique that may be ready more quickly is the use of adjuvants, or substances that would be included in the vaccine solution to reduce the actual dose of vaccine protein material required to stimulate an effective immune response in the recipient. The use of an adjuvant would increase the number of people who could receive vaccine out of a certain production capacity, so fewer eggs would be needed. Currently, 300 million doses of influenza vaccine are produced yearly worldwide, with a maximum manufacturing capacity of about 1 billion doses per year.[11]

WHO GETS THE VACCINE?

Vaccines will be distributed according to a defined priority list. Since a vaccine may not have undergone the usual full process of development, its effectiveness and side effects will have to be closely monitored.

Initially, there will be limited amounts of vaccine. In Canada, we are very fortunate that our contract vaccine supplier, ID Biomedical (now part of the conglomerate GlaxoSmithKline), has a production capacity of up to 8 million doses of vaccine per month. You will probably need two shots, a month apart, to induce a good "immunological memory." Public health agencies will probably organize mass clinics in each community for this purpose.

Most pandemic plans, including the Canadian and U.S. plans, have a defined priority list determining the order in which people are to receive vaccine.[12-13] The goals of these lists are to preserve services essential for all members of the public and to protect those who are most susceptible to serious complications of influenza infection. The priority list may be revised as pandemic conditions and issues change, and as data emerge upon patterns of illness. As of March 2006, the Canadian priority list for vaccination includes:[12]

- **Health care workers (about 600,000):** nurses, physicians, respiratory therapists, paramedics, and public health workers.

Health care and public health will be the front line of
defence in a pandemic. The workers need to be protected in
order to protect and care for everyone else.

- **Essential service workers (about 1 million):** fire, police,
utility workers (gas, electricity, water), public transport workers, essential goods transport workers, vaccine manufacturing
workers. Essential service workers must ensure that public
safety, essential utilities, and the distribution of essential
goods are minimally interrupted.

- **Persons at high risk for complications from influenza:**
persons older than 65 years of age, children between 6 and
23 months of age, persons with high-risk medical conditions.[12]

Demographic priorities will probably be revisited as
data emerge during a pandemic. Elsewhere we have
discussed the "age signature" of influenza pandemics.
Although young adults are often affected by influenza
pandemics to an unusually greater degree than they
are affected by seasonal influenza, the current
Canadian priority list recognizes that older people
may still experience a higher absolute risk of ill consequences, even if the degree to which they are affected
is closer to their usual pattern in seasonal influenza.
As the pandemic plays out, we will see if an "age signature" is demonstrated.

There will be a great deal of ongoing surveillance and
research concerning the vaccine and those who have
received it, as it is being administered to the first groups
of people on the priority list and then to the general
public. If circumstances warrant it, the vaccine may be
used before it has undergone the usual comprehensive
testing.

TO VACCINATE OR NOT?

The decision to embark upon a vaccination campaign may be a difficult judgment, weighing the damage caused by a pandemic as well as what is known and unknown about a new vaccine.

In a perfect world, every medical treatment would be perfectly effective, have no side effects, and be fully tested and understood. These things are not the case at the best of times, and the world is not perfect. All new medical treatments are tested to demonstrate that they are sufficiently effective and beneficial, that their common side effects are well known and that all major side effects are reasonable in light of the benefits they provide. Despite this testing, after a new pill or vaccine is brought into general use, sometimes new side effects are discovered. What's more, the choice of certain treatments hinges upon the dangers within a situation. Some treatments for heart attacks have serious potential risks. It would not be a good idea to give them to someone who is not having a heart attack, because there's no reason for that person to take those risks. However, for someone who is having a heart attack, the potential benefits of such inherently risky treatments may greatly outweigh the risks that are involved.

An influenza pandemic creates a comparable situation at the level of a population. Even during a pandemic, no vaccine will be used until there is reasonable scientific evidence that it is effective, and that the potential side effects are reasonably outweighed by the risks posed by a pandemic. However, what is "reasonable" depends to a great degree upon the situation during a pandemic. If the pandemic progresses rapidly with many deaths, it is more reasonable to proceed with vaccination of a population at an earlier stage of scientific development, so long as the known benefits of a vaccine, clearly assessed, outweigh what is known about its possible side effects and the damage done by the pandemic. If the pandemic moves very slowly while killing very few people, it behooves scientists to more fully assess the vaccine before mass immunization. In this scenario, public health decision-makers will want to tolerate only the typical minute acceptable risks of side effects from vaccination, before embarking upon widespread immunization. These decisions must be based upon science and data, but they also entail exceedingly difficult judgment calls.

During the swine flu episode in 1976 in the United States, a widespread vaccination campaign was undertaken because of the assessment that there was a substantial pandemic risk to the general population, and that similar influenza vaccines were known to be safe. Canadians were immunized with the same vaccine. The pandemic did not materialize. There was a suggestion that the swine flu vaccine increased the incidence of Guillain-Barré syndrome, a neurological condition that occurs with often unknown causes regardless of vaccination. This was not proven but was one of the reasons that the vaccination campaign was halted.

In retrospect, it is easy to criticize the swine flu immunization campaign. Some point to this campaign as one of the contributing reasons that strong anti-vaccine opinions exist in some quarters. However, many public health observers still believe that, given the knowledge and information available at that time, the right decisions were made. If a worldwide pandemic had materialized, and a vaccination had significantly protected its recipients from serious illness and death, there would have been little criticism of the decision to immunize. Even if there had been good proof of a small number of serious side effects such as Guillain-Barré syndrome resulting from swine flu immunization, we would probably have accepted that the benefits of such vaccination had outweighed its side effects. As Dr. Arthur Silverstein, a virologist and former adviser to the U.S. Senate Health Committee during the swine flu episode in 1976, put it during a 1983 CBC interview, "It was justified in this respect: that the scientists, based on what they then knew about influenza virus and influenza disease . . . had every right to expect that there was a fairly good probability that a dangerous influenza pandemic would sweep the world, and there was time to get ready and practise preventive medicine."[14]

One of the criticisms of the swine flu immunization campaign is that it proceeded in the fall of 1976, even when it did not seem that the risks identified in the spring of 1976 were clearly advancing. The theoretical concern regarding a pandemic still existed, but there were not further clear signals that we were getting closer to the brink of a full pandemic. Some suggest that we would not act in the same way today without such indications. The American public health authorities used the best science that was available and understood in 1976. We believe that we now know more, but of course our science always risks being viewed as incomplete, in retrospect. As Dr. Silverstein put it, "We have learned some valuable lessons, at least I hope we have . . . from the '76 affair. One of the lessons is that we can do it [a widespread immunization campaign], but we have to take a little more care of the progression of events . . . There have to be points at which one stops: if the flu doesn't come back, if it's not that serious, if it does not kill, if it is going to be benign. There have to be clear signals about when to proceed and when to start immunizing."[14]

Other criticisms of the 1976 swine flu event are political, contending that political momentum helped propel the immunization campaign forward once millions of dollars had been committed to it. This highlights the reality that public health and policy decisions are never pure science but take place in a complex atmosphere of social goals and fears, as well as political ones.

A key problem is that no one can predict the future. They couldn't do so in 1976, and neither can we. Public health decision-making about whether to fast-track the production and distribution of a new vaccine, or take any other measures with potential risks and costs, must use the best available scientific information and tolerate some degree of the unknown. The best possible judgments must be made in the interest of the public, but in retrospect some of them may not look like the right decisions. This must be accepted from the outset.

The swine flu immunization campaign was undertaken when the situation was, according to our more recently developed classification system, at Phase 5. Regarding the next pandemic threat, difficult decisions may have to be made whether to intervene with vaccination during a similar stage of risk. This question will arise if time and advances in vaccine technology give us an effective H5N1 vaccine while H5N1 evolves further ability to transmit from human to human but before it has ignited a full-blown pandemic. Acting earlier might serve to better prevent illness and death, but it might mean that less is known about the trade-off between the risks and benefits of an immunization campaign.

If H5N1 rapidly develops the ability to transmit from human to human before vaccine technology and production capacity advance appreciably from their present state, final vaccine development can begin only at the start of Phase 6. We will probably not have the opportunity to embark upon widespread immunization of populations of people until Phase 6 of the pandemic, and very possibly not until Phase 6 is well under way. There may be no vaccine available until the second wave of the pandemic, highlighting the importance of public health containment measures in the meantime.

Even if a vaccine can be produced rapidly at the outset of Phase 6 of a pandemic, if currently limited worldwide production capacity is unchanged, most of the world will not receive vaccine in a timely fashion. Once we have reached that point, the consequences of an influenza pandemic for a population will be better known, and the trade-off of the vaccine's benefits and risks will be clearer, but it will be too late for most to benefit from this knowledge.

CHAPTER 12

THE TRUTH ABOUT ANTIVIRAL MEDICATIONS

THIS CHAPTER IN ONE PAGE . . .

- **Tamiflu (oseltamivir) and Relenza (zanimivir) are currently the antiviral medications of choice for seasonal and pandemic influenza. The data exist for seasonal influenza, and the inference is made that these drugs will be useful during the pandemic.**

- **For treatment of seasonal influenza illness, Tamiflu and Relenza, if taken within the first 36 to 48 hours of symptoms, shorten the average length of illness by one to two days. They decrease complications such as pneumonia and hospitalization by 30% to 60%. It is not clear whether they improve survival rates in people who would die from influenza infection.**

- **For prevention of seasonal influenza, if taken daily, antivirals decrease the risk of illness by 70% to 90%.**

- **Data for the effectiveness of these medications in treating H5N1 or other future pandemics are mostly at a laboratory or theoretical level and are limited. We must be wary of the possible development of drug resistance.**

- **Improper use of antiviral medications may favour the development of resistant viral strains.**

- **Governments plan to use antiviral medications as one of many public health strategies to mitigate the pandemic's effect on society.**

- **Deciding whether to personally stockpile these medications ahead of an unknown pandemic is not easy. There are both advantages and disadvantages to doing so.**

ANTIVIRAL MEDICATIONS FOR INFLUENZA

Much media attention has focused recently on influenza antiviral medications, particularly Tamiflu. Popular news has covered government stockpiling of this medication, personal stockpiling of this medication, the relative worldwide "shortage" of Tamiflu, and the notion that it will be an effective treatment for the pandemic strain of influenza, but one that is in short supply. As physicians, we are commonly asked: "Is Tamiflu going to work during a pandemic? Should I buy some now?"

Antiviral medications can play a useful role as part of a coordinated public health strategy to respond to pandemic influenza. They also have potential benefits for individual people. They are not a panacea. As with any medications, their use can be accompanied by side effects and complications. There are currently four main antivirals for treatment of influenza infections. The older ones, Amantadine and Rimantadine, are part of a class called adamantanes. The newer drugs, Tamiflu and Relenza, are in a class called neuraminidase inhibitors.

The older drugs have more potential serious side effects and have been associated with the rapid emergence of drug-resistant influenza strains. If drug-resistant influenza strains are created, they can be transmitted to others, and those persons' infections will no longer be treatable by those drugs. The older drugs are cheap, at about 50 cents per day of treatment, versus about $10 per day for the newer drugs. They have been around for 30 years and were used to some good effect during the 1968–69 influenza pandemic. Nonetheless, they are really not a good choice in comparison with the newer drugs and are no longer recommended for routine use in seasonal influenza. They are unlikely to have a role in an influenza pandemic.[1-2]

Tamiflu and Relenza are now the primary antiviral medications used for influenza, both in seasonal infections and for the anticipated pandemic strain. Each drug has advantages and disadvantages. Tamiflu comes in both pill and liquid form, while Relenza comes only as a dry powder and can be taken only by inhalation, much like some asthma medications. The inhaled route of delivery of Relenza means that it cannot be used by people with asthma or chronic obstructive pulmonary disease since it may exacerbate those problems. Neither drug comes in an intravenous formulation, which is relevant because sometimes the sickest people can be given only intravenous medications.

Tamiflu can treat influenza not only in the lung but also in the blood and other parts of the body, making it more useful in widespread influenza infection. Relenza acts primarily on the lungs and has little action on other systems in the body. However, this characteristic may give it some advantages for use in people in whom it is important to avoid other interactions in the body, and for pregnant women, since the side effects of these newer antivirals upon fetal development are not known. Tamiflu can be used in children at least one year old, while Relenza can be used only in children who are at least seven years old.

TREATING INFLUENZA ILLNESS: THE SCIENCE

There is strong scientific evidence showing that otherwise healthy adults with seasonal influenza who take Relenza or Tamiflu within 36 to 48 hours after the start of influenza symptoms get better about one to two days faster.[3] There is some evidence that Tamiflu decreases seasonal-influenza-related complications such as pneumonia and lowers hospitalizations by about 30% to 60%.[4] There are no data proving that these drugs reduce the death rate in people who become seriously ill from seasonal influenza.

No clear data show us how effective these drugs are in the occasional human cases of the H5N1 strain that have occurred, although these drugs have been used to treat these illnesses. The human cases of H5N1 have been few up to this point and have occurred sporadically in different countries, making it hard to collect scientific information to assess treatment in a standardized and meaningful way. In a laboratory setting, and in animals, preliminary studies show promise that Tamiflu and Relenza can prevent the H5N1 virus from replicating, leading us to be hopeful that they should have some effect in treating human H5N1 infection.[5-7] Note that these particular studies have been done largely by scientists who are in one way or another associated with, funded, or paid by the pharmaceutical companies that manufacture these drugs. This is not unusual in the drug industry. Remember that we cannot be certain that the next influenza pandemic will be caused by a derivative of the H5N1 strain.

These drugs are certainly the most potentially useful class of medications that exist for treating illness associated with a possible influenza pandemic. However, their precise degree of usefulness in treating current H5N1 infection or any future pandemic strain of influenza is not known. It will be further clarified as we gain more experience in using them during a pandemic.

When neuraminidase inhibitors are given to people either before or shortly after they are exposed to someone with influenza, as a treatment to prevent seasonal influenza illness, their effectiveness is more impressive.[8-12] This is called a prophylactic use of medication, or a preventive treatment, because the people are not yet infected. In healthy adults, both Tamiflu and Relenza are about 70% to 90% effective in preventing seasonal influenza. There is also some evidence that they are effective for prevention in children and elderly people.

People who are taking neuraminidase inhibitors for prevention are still at risk of being infected by the virus. However, if infected, the drug may prevent the virus from producing symptoms and illness in their bodies. This is called an asymptomatic infection. To complicate matters, it is unknown whether asymptomatic infection allows an infected person to develop immunity to that strain of influenza. Therefore, it is unknown whether such a person who stops preventive treatment will fall ill if exposed to the same virus again.

We have no data regarding the effectiveness of these drugs in preventive treatment against H5N1 infection. At the time of this writing, H5N1 only occasionally spreads from animals to humans, and very rarely from human to human, so it is not possible to collect any data on the specific role of these drugs in preventing human-to-human spread. The current thinking is that Tamiflu and Relenza should be effective in this role. Tamiflu is being used as a preventive treatment for close contacts of persons or birds ill with H5N1, such as family contacts, health care workers, and poultry farmers. The older drugs are not thought to have as useful a role in this regard, largely because of drug resistance. We also have no scientific data showing safety of the use of Tamiflu over the months, or even years, that one would have to regularly take it if one wished to use it as preventive treatment for the duration of a pandemic.

DRUG RESISTANCE

Sometimes an infectious agent like a bacteria or a virus can develop the ability to evade an antibiotic or an antiviral medication that is meant to stop its survival and reproduction. This is called drug resistance. It often happens after an infectious agent has been treated with such a medication and, over time, has opportunities to adapt itself to fight the drug through a process of genetic change. If viral resistance to Relenza or Tamiflu develops and becomes widespread, its usefulness in both treatment and prevention will be decreased.

Even though there has been a very low rate of resistance to these newer drugs, the possibility of viral resistance developing is a concern. There has already been a report of drug resistance in two patients with H5N1 influenza infection who were treated with Tamiflu in Vietnam.[14] It is difficult to predict if and when widespread resistance to these drugs will occur in H5N1 or any other strain of influenza. However, with trillions of copies of influenza viruses circulating around the world and undergoing constant genetic changes, resistance to any single antiviral medication is a very real possibility.

In the event that resistance develops to one of these drugs, at least we have the other one, but they are both from the same family of antivirals. So it is conceivable that once resistance to one of them develops, resistance to the other drug could quickly follow. We should continue to develop new antivirals, as well as make plans to use the current medications rationally and carefully, in order to minimize the risk of resistance developing.

One of the major concerns with personal stockpiling of antiviral medications is that without professional guidance, people may use them inappropriately. Our experience with antibiotic and other antiviral medications tells us that, as a general principle, when such drugs are used inappropriately, whether in too small a dose for a given situation or for an insufficient length of time, this can increase the risk that resistance to the medication will develop. There is a substantial literature that shows us that even when drugs are prescribed for a specific ongoing medical condition, people often don't use them appropriately; people often insist upon antibiotics when they don't need them, or, when prescribed antibiotics, they stop taking them early once they feel better and end up not finishing the treatment course. People miss doses of medications or share them with their family members and friends. Any medication, including antiviral drugs, should be used for a defined situation, and in a particular dose for a specified length of time. Usage of antiviral medications outside of well-considered parameters may favour the development of antiviral resistance.

More widespread use of a medication, even correctly, can also increase the chance of resistance developing. It's possible that if people who are destined to recover from their influenza use a drug like Tamiflu widely, this may promote resistance, rendering the drug resistant and ineffective in people whose lives could otherwise be saved by it. The difficulties with this suggestion are that no one can predict in advance who is destined to recover, and we don't really have strong scientific evidence that Tamiflu saves lives anyway once people become ill with influenza.

THE "SHORTAGE" OF TAMIFLU

The pharmaceutical company Roche produces Tamiflu. Late in 2005, because of a shortage, Roche announced that it was going to suspend sales of Tamiflu to individuals in Canada in order to focus on institutional orders. In the spring of 2006, it announced that it would once again make the drug available for retail purchases while continuing to fill government orders. We think it's worth pointing out that over time, the "shortage" of Tamiflu and other antiviral medications is a self-correcting "problem." Before the upsurge in world interest in the drug, Tamiflu as a treatment for seasonal influenza was somewhat of a commercial disappointment to Roche, with the only country using it to an appreciable degree being Japan.

It is largely being bought by governments for pandemic stockpiling purposes, meaning that these supplies are mostly not being consumed. Once institutional orders are filled, Roche, like any drug company, will be motivated to continue sales of its products, including sales to individuals. So it's somewhat incorrect to view government stockpiling as taking place *instead* of individual stockpiling. It's probably more correct to take the view that the opportunity for governments to stockpile has been given priority ahead of the opportunity for individuals to purchase these medications.

INTELLECTUAL PROPERTY ISSUES IN THE PHARMACEUTICAL INDUSTRY

In view of the current climate of anxiety about a possible influenza pandemic, many governments and people are eager to obtain Tamiflu. Roche says the production of this drug involves a multi-step, complicated process that takes six to eight months after the raw materials are in hand, and that the supply of raw materials is limited. Apparently, one part of the process involves a step that can lead to explosions. Others in the pharmaceutical industry contend that the manufacture process is not significantly more complicated than for other drugs. One of the active ingredients in Tamiflu, shikimic acid, is found mainly in the star anise plant, whose primary source is in China. Chemists have managed to produce synthetic shikimic acid, and the use of this technique to produce base material for Tamiflu production is being explored.

Gilead Sciences, the company that initially developed Tamiflu and sold the licence to Roche in 1996, informed Roche in June 2005 that it was terminating the 1996 agreement giving Roche the rights to make and sell Tamiflu.[15] Gilead cited "ongoing neglect of the product" for the past five years. Gilead's chief executive, John Martin, said at the time, "Roche has not adequately demonstrated the requisite commitment to Tamiflu since its launch in the United States nearly six years ago, nor has it allocated the necessary resources to realize the potential of the product as a treatment and a preventative for influenza." Tamiflu was, in fact, a poor seller until concerns regarding a possible influenza pandemic began to mount in 2003. In the first business quarter of 2005, Tamiflu sales by Roche quadrupled to $330 million, and both Roche and Gilead have now, not surprisingly, come to a renegotiated agreement.[16]

Meanwhile, a number of countries are developing their own capability to produce generic Tamiflu. In

November 2005, Vietnam was granted permission by Roche to produce a generic version of the drug, and other countries such as China, India, Taiwan, and Thailand are reportedly either going ahead with production or in discussion with Roche for a sublicence. It is expected that generic versions of Tamiflu will be available late in 2006. The issue of intellectual property surrounding pharmaceuticals is an important one. Some argue that the imperative of a pandemic threat justifies ignoring standard patent protections such as the ones that Roche holds for Tamiflu. Cipla, an Indian drug manufacturer, announced in late 2005 that it would produce Tamiflu as a generic drug with or without the permission of Roche. "Right or wrong, we're going to commercialize and make Tamiflu," Dr. Yusuf K. Hamied, chairman of Cipla, told the *New York Times* on October 14, 2005.[17]

One danger in ignoring patents is that it greatly reduces the incentive for any drug manufacturer to develop new medications. At present, we have only two antiviral medications that will probably play a role in managing the next pandemic, and the development of drug resistance is a very real concern. It would be preferable to have a wide range of antiviral medications that are potentially effective against influenza. If pharmaceutical patent protections are widely ignored, there is little motivation for such companies to undertake the lengthy and expensive process of developing and producing other potentially useful drugs—which we would very much like to have available in the event of a pandemic.

GOVERNMENT STRATEGIES FOR STOCKPILING AND USE OF ANTIVIRALS

Since the worldwide avian H5N1 outbreak started in 2003, and as public attention has grown surrounding this issue, governments, institutions, and individuals have been stockpiling antivirals, largely Tamiflu, for potential pandemic use. At the time of this writing, there is a worldwide "shortage" created by the recent influx of orders for Tamiflu, and a 12-to-18-month waiting list for large government and institutional orders

The way in which these supplies will be used as part of a public health strategy will depend upon the pandemic phase and the specific issues that arise, and it is discussed more fully elsewhere in this book. In Phases 4 and 5, these drugs may be used to treat illness, and to preventively treat all contacts of people who have become ill from a novel strain of influenza. At that point, they may also be used as part of a focused, WHO-directed containment strategy in the geographic area that first experiences significant human-to-human transmission of a novel strain of influenza. Such a strategy may involve aggressively treating everyone within the area, if the outbreak is localized there. The goal will be to delay or avert a pandemic, and the successful implementation of this strategy would obviously benefit all citizens of the world. Individual countries may act similarly within their borders.

In Phase 6, it is unlikely that government strategies will involve treating all contacts preventively, or treating all those who become ill with influenza. Instead, there will be a shift toward groups of people who are defined as priority groups to receive medication, with an eye toward maximizing the benefits that antiviral medications deliver to society during the pandemic.

The WHO and other experts have recommended that governments stockpile enough antiviral medication to treat 25% of their population, with about 90% of the stockpile being Tamiflu and 10% being Relenza. Canada and the United States have currently outlined priority groups for access to these antivirals, as do most pandemic plans. These priority groups include people who are judged to be at particularly high risk of serious illness and death from illness, and people who are felt to be essential to the functioning of society during a pandemic.

As more understanding of the disease and the utility of treatment emerges, the priority groups and their order may change. The definition of "high risk" may change, depending on how the pandemic is seen to affect the population. For example, if it causes more harm in young children than in other groups, they may be classified as high-risk. Even if there is a shortage of antivirals, medications will not be strictly reserved for the first priority group, then the second, the third, and so on. Antivirals will be distributed to most priority groups, but in greater proportion to the higher priority groups. Having priority groups in the Canadian Pandemic Plan has been controversial and is fraught with ethical dilemmas. Consequently, there is a current consideration to abolish this list of priority groups.

Some groups such as essential service workers and health care workers have been identified in the priority list for preventive treatment. This is to ensure that society continues to function through the course of a pandemic, and that those who care for people who are ill can continue to do so. In the case of health care workers, this position also recognizes the reality that they will be working closely with people who have influenza. At present, governments are not generally stockpiling enough to provide preventive treatment for every citizen.

Current Canadian Pandemic Plan Priority List[18]

These are the official priorities for allocation of treatment resources, in descending order, as of March 2006. However, there is currently a reconsideration of having any priority list because of the ethical dilemmas it poses.

1. Treatment of persons hospitalized for influenza.
2. Treatment of ill health care and emergency services workers.
3. Treatment of ill high-risk persons in the community.
4. Preventive treatment of health care workers.
5. Control of outbreaks in high-risk residents of institutions (nursing homes and other chronic care facilities).
6. Preventive treatment of essential service workers.
7. Preventive treatment of high-risk persons hospitalized for illnesses other than influenza.
8. Preventive treatment of high-risk persons in the community.

The stockpiling of medications by governments has been met with some criticism for a variety of reasons. Public costs are an issue, especially when many health systems around the world already have difficulty allocating a limited amount of resources to immediate health issues. Dr. Richard Schabas, a former chief medical officer of health for the province of Ontario, pointed out in a *Globe and Mail* article on March 20, 2006, that the proposed expenditure of $25 million by Ontario hospitals on Tamiflu in that year is an amount sufficient to employ 300 nurses. The memory of the past and the fear of the unknown have significant effects on human behaviour. Health care workers in Ontario have been forever changed by the mental and physical challenges and the damage done by SARS, and are wary of what the future holds for them at their place of work. This is reflected in ongoing lawsuits by some health care workers, who accuse institutions of not doing enough to protect them from SARS in hospitals during that outbreak. It is in this context that many hospitals have decided to stockpile Tamiflu as preventive therapy for their staff in the event a pandemic arrives. There is a concern that without the extra protection of Tamiflu, some health care workers will not show up for work, thereby jeopardizing patient care.

In jurisdictions in which public sale of Tamiflu was suspended in order to fill orders from governments, some feel that individual people should be allowed to purchase the drug to "protect themselves" and that this option should not be inhibited by government purchasing. Other observers feel that government stockpiling may inhibit people's access to Tamiflu in a timely fashion. A molecular biologist in Canberra, Graeme Laver, said in the *Australian* on March 1, 2006, "Tamiflu should be available in every chemist in the country, without a prescription, so you can get it in time."[19] Unscrupulous profiteers have been selling oseltamivir by mail or through the Internet, sometimes at up to $20 per pill. There is price gouging, and some have been selling fake pills.[20]

PERSONAL STOCKPILING OF ANTIVIRAL MEDICATIONS

At some point soon, government and institutional orders for antivirals will be filled, and drugs like Tamiflu will again be readily available to the general public. We cannot predict the timing of a pandemic, but it is statistically unlikely that it will begin within the relatively short period of time that will be necessary for governments to have their orders filled for Tamiflu. Therefore antiviral drugs will soon be back in abundance on the shelves, if they aren't already, making it theoretically easier for people who want a personal stockpile of antiviral medications to acquire one. Should you have such a supply for yourself and your family? There is no easy answer to this question.

Dr. Lam's Perspective
Antiviral Stockpiling and the Doctor–Patient Relationship

Physicians are now commonly asked for prescriptions for Tamiflu by people who wish to stockpile this medication. As physicians, our mandate is to help patients protect and improve their health, and it's always much easier and more pleasant to do what people ask us to do. But the doctor-patient relationship has, as a core value, our obligation to assess a patient's present condition and make a recommendation. If physicians feel that a treatment is not necessary or not beneficial, or may in fact be harmful, their obligation to refuse this treatment is just as strong as their obligation would be to give a treatment to someone when they feel it is beneficial. Our responsibility is to consider a situation and make this judgment, not simply to write prescriptions.

It is much more personally and professionally difficult to say no to a patient who requests something that I believe to be unwise. Refusing a request consumes time and energy, often by way of conflict. Frankly, it's easier to acquiesce. When we say no, it is because we have strongly held professional reasons for doing so. As physicians, we are also sometimes subject to the tempting appeal of "doing something," even if we truly believe that doing nothing is actually the better choice. So if you ask your doctor for something, whether it is an antibiotic, Tamiflu, or some other treatment, and she is spending a significant amount of time trying to explain to you why she will not do this, you at least should realize that she is usually creating work for herself by refusing, and doing this out of a profound belief that it's "not the right thing."

Tamiflu stockpiling is conceptually tricky, because to prescribe this drug for stockpiles is to prescribe a drug that will possibly be helpful for a pandemic strain of influenza but has not yet proven to be, for a pandemic that has not yet occurred and whose timing is highly unpredictable, to treat people who are not yet sick. In addition, there are important concerns that inappropriate use of antiviral medications may lead to unnecessary side effects and the development of resistant strains of virus during a pandemic, further jeopardizing public health.

REASONS TO HAVE A PERSONAL STOCKPILE OF ANTIVIRAL MEDICATIONS

It may work: In seasonal influenza, the newer antiviral medications are somewhat effective when used for treatment and more effective for prevention. The more scientifically supported way to use the antiviral medications is for prevention, although this requires a large number of pills. For prevention, you would want to buy enough for the first Phase 6 pandemic wave, which is expected to last six to eight weeks, hoping that a vaccine will be available for the second wave.

On the other hand . . . : Remember that the data we have are only for seasonal influenza, and at present we are inferring that they will be applicable to a pandemic strain of influenza. These data are sufficiently convincing for governments to have decided to stockpile medications, but you should realize that there are no guarantees concerning the usefulness of Tamiflu in a pandemic.

It's in short supply: One motivation for personal stockpiling is the feeling that there is a shortage of antiviral medications, and that there may be limited supplies when the pandemic arrives. A pandemic will cause a sudden increase in the number of people who become ill with influenza and in the prevalence of serious influenza illness. One fear is that demand for antiviral medications may be greater than immediate supply. It is also understood that these medications need to be started quickly after the onset of symptoms in order to be effective. No one can say when a pandemic will occur.

On the other hand ... : The "shortage" is probably temporary, created primarily by the upsurge in interest in bird flu and this product. Roche is increasing production capacity, and other companies may be starting to produce generic versions in late 2006. There is the possibility of other new medications being developed, especially now with increased market potential for such medications. There may be plenty available at a much lower price within the next little while. No one knows whether a pandemic will come before that happens, but there is a statistically good chance that it won't.

You're not confident that your government will provide for you: You may have read the priority lists and realized that you do not fit into any of the priority categories. Your assessment may be that if you are not on a government priority list, the only way to ensure that you will receive

antiviral medication that might benefit you is to provide it for yourself. This sentiment is understandable.
Although intellectually you may agree that the use of
antiviral medications for the maximum societal benefit
is admirable, you may still want to take steps to ensure
supply for yourself if this has some possibility of bene-
fiting you. You may also take the view that having your
own personal supply of antiviral medications will mean
one less person for whom your government has to provide drugs in the event of a pandemic.

On the other hand . . . : For the population of a country,
these drugs are likely to do the greatest good as part of a
coordinated public health strategy. Remember that the
priority lists are written as a starting point and are meant
to be adjusted during a pandemic as needed. If your age
group turns out to have an unusually high death rate,
you may find yourself in a priority group. If there is a
limited supply of drug in relation to demand, there is a
strong ethical argument that this supply should be
directed by governments for the greatest societal benefit.
This is presently true, although, as discussed above, we
believe that this will be a temporary situation.

Reasons to Not Have a Personal Stockpile
of Antiviral Medications

It's expensive: Each tablet of Tamiflu costs at least $5.
Preventive treatment requires one tablet a day, and it
would be sensible to use preventive treatment for the duration of a six-to-eight-week pandemic wave, let's say for 50
days. A 50-day course would cost about $250 per person.
You can't take less than this or share it between people at
a lower dose, because this will compromise its effectiveness
in you, in addition to increasing the probability of causing

resistance to develop. Treatment requires at least two tablets daily for five days. A treatment course of five days would cost $50 per person, but there are fewer data for effectiveness in treating illness than for prevention.

On the other hand . . . : If it actually prevents you from catching pandemic influenza, or helps you to recover, that's hard to put a dollar figure on. You probably would have gotten better anyhow, but there's a small chance that you might have become seriously ill or died. Many people spend much more money on far more foolish things. As time goes on, influenza drugs may become cheaper due to competition and the development of new or generic drugs.

It's not fair: Since the cost of Tamiflu is prohibitive, many people don't have the spare cash to buy a Tamiflu stockpile. The authors believe that health is a basic human right, and from this follows the notion that people's ability to get a health resource should be predicated upon the need for that resource, and not upon wealth.

On the other hand . . . : Although Canada provides universal access to health care, it does not provide universal coverage for pharmaceuticals. Some may argue that it should, but it doesn't, so people with more money already have better access to expensive drugs. Better access to Tamiflu is one example.

The shelf life is only five years, and then it may expire, become useless, and be a waste of money: The pandemic may not come during the shelf life of your Tamiflu stockpile. If further resistance develops, the effectiveness of Tamiflu may be limited. Superior medications may be developed in the future. If you have a limited amount of money to spend on preparedness, there may be more useful things to spend it on. We would suggest that some of the preparations previously discussed for general emergency preparedness, in ways that would be useful for any disaster, might be better ways to spend your money. Tamiflu won't keep you warm during an ice storm.

On the other hand . . . : Tamiflu is the drug we've got now. It's not our business to tell you what to spend your money on. People spend money on sillier things.

Resistance may develop: Using these drugs inappropriately might favour the development of resistant strains of the novel influenza.

On the other hand . . . : You may make a strong personal commitment to educating yourself about influenza, and to using your personal stockpile only in a rational and well-informed way guided by medical advice. In any case, even using these drugs appropriately may contribute to the development of resistance, given the likely widespread use of these drugs during a pandemic, and the tendency of the influenza virus to mutate.

> If you do decide to stockpile antiviral medications, here are our suggestions for responsible use.
>
> • Have a discussion with your family physician about these issues, understanding that he is under no obligation to provide such a prescription for you. In fact, for him to do so is somewhat out of keeping with what a physician usually does.
>
> • If you do purchase a stockpile, think clearly in advance about how you're going to use it—whether for preventive treatment or treatment of illness. Think about who in your family will be treated. Remember

that you should not take half doses or treatment courses shorter than recommended.

- Educate yourself so that you know when to use your stockpile. If you plan to use your stockpile for preventive treatment, have a discussion with your physician about when this would be appropriate. If you plan to use it for treatment if you develop influenza, learn about the symptoms of influenza so that you will know when you probably have it.

- Even if you have drugs in your medicine cabinet, it would be useful to speak with a health professional before you start to take them.

There is no absolute answer about whether you should have a personal stockpile. The restricted availability of antiviral medications limits this option at present, but this will probably change eventually. At present, there is no Canadian professional guideline for physicians on whether to provide prescriptions for such stockpiles. In the absence of such guidelines, once public sales resume (as they probably will have by the time you read this), the issue of stockpiling antivirals remains a matter between you and your physician. If you decide to speak to your physician about having a personal stockpile of antiviral medications, she may have some very good and valid reasons for discouraging you, or she may provide a prescription to you after some discussion.

We certainly don't believe that the stockpiling of Tamiflu by individual or national governments is the central issue of pandemic preparedness. The drug is a legitimate, possibly useful resource in a pandemic. It may have captured an unusual amount of public attention because of our collective fascination with pills; our culture is very interested in the power, real or otherwise, of "things." Our devotion of this much space to exploring the issue is a reflection of the fact that we see a great deal of interest in the topic, which therefore merits a full discussion of some of its parameters. Neither the authors nor our family members have personal stockpiles of these medications.

CHAPTER 13

IT'S NOT SO SIMPLE: ETHICAL DILEMMAS DURING AN INFLUENZA PANDEMIC

THIS CHAPTER IN ONE PAGE . . .

- Individual people from all walks of life, health care professionals, public health officials, and people in government may face many ethical dilemmas in the course of a pandemic.
- Some issues with important ethical parameters are:
  - When and how to isolate and quarantine citizens who have fallen ill or have been exposed to the pandemic strain of influenza, while respecting personal liberties as much as possible.
  - How to ensure that health care workers are able and willing to work, despite the increased occupational hazards of working with influenza-stricken patients.
  - How to ration scarce health care resources such as medications, vaccines, and advanced medical equipment, such as life-saving ventilators.
  - How to balance global and local priorities, which may sometimes be different.

DIFFICULT DECISIONS AND ETHICAL CONFLICTS

The specific decisions that must be made and the practical implementation of those decisions during a pandemic, are inherently difficult. They must be informed by an understanding of the scientific and technical issues surrounding pandemic influenza and the possible measures to address it. At their core, these decisions often embody serious ethical dilemmas.

What circumstances give society the right to limit the freedom of individuals by imposing isolation or quarantine? Is it the duty of health care workers to report to their posts if this work increases their risk of contracting influenza and may affect their families? When resources such as antiviral medications, specialized medical equipment, or vaccinations are limited, who gets them first? When global health organizations such as the WHO advise national or regional authorities on what to do, how do authorities decide about actions that are good for the globe but create problems for people in their region? We know that our current understanding of the upcoming pandemic is incomplete and that during the pandemic there will be an ongoing process of data gathering and analysis, so how do we approach decisions that must be made immediately in the face of such a changeable and incomplete science?

Good governments will need to be honest and make public the rationale behind difficult decisions that affect people's freedoms and their chances of surviving the pandemic. Often there won't be a single "right" decision, because authorities will need to consider not only incomplete scientific information about the pandemic virus, but also the goals that are desired and society's values and priorities. Governments and leaders must make a serious commitment to open public communication of available scientific information, as well as the goals and rationales behind difficult choices. This is the responsibility that is placed in the hands of governments, and this kind of honesty is necessary in order to maintain the trust of society and counter the ill effects of a pandemic.

This chapter outlines the central ethical dilemmas that are expected to arise, and some of the associated problems. We are not able to give the "final word" on these issues, but there is value in considering them.

LIMITS ON FREEDOM

What right does society have to impose isolation or quarantine, or otherwise limit the freedoms of individual people?

Quarantine, isolation, and travel restrictions impinge upon individuals' freedoms of movement and rights of assembly. Contact tracing and contact management may conflict with people's right to privacy. Most societies accept these measures within certain parameters if they are necessary to protect society from infectious disease. Public health legislation such as Ontario's Health Protection and Promotion Act[2] provides legal mechanisms to undertake and, if necessary, enforce some of these measures. A federal act makes it legally possible to isolate and quarantine people at Canadian points of international entry and exit.[3] There are current parallels in use: for instance, people with infectious tuberculosis who refuse to be treated for this condition can be detained to decrease the risk of transmission to the public.

During the SARS crisis, over 23,000 persons were

quarantined in Toronto.[4] Public health staff asked people to stay home for up to 10 days and provided support and monitoring by telephone. In only 27 cases was a written order mandating quarantine issued under Ontario's Health Protection and Promotion Act.[4] Later research showed that most people who were quarantined accepted this situation as a form of civic duty, although they had legitimate concerns about lost income and job security.[5]

Society has obligations to people who are isolated or quarantined. If people are willing to have their freedom restricted for the good of society, it is reasonable to expect that society will ensure that they have enough food and provisions, that they don't suffer financial hardship as a result of isolation or quarantine, and that their jobs are protected when they are able to return to work. At a practical level, pandemic planning for isolation and quarantine needs to include consideration of who will buy and deliver food to people who can't leave the house, how they will pay their bills and send their mail, and who will provide some funds in lieu of lost income. These kinds of details are essential if such measures are to be fair and successful.

One problem is the lack of good scientific evidence from past pandemics showing that the isolation and quarantine of individual people altered the broad course of pandemics. The practical and ethical problem is this: given that isolation and quarantine will clearly affect the freedoms of individuals and have economic costs for both individuals and society, it's easier to judge whether these costs are worthwhile if we have clear scientific guidance about their usefulness. Note that during the 1918–19 pandemic, these measures were implemented only in Phase 6. In contrast, current planning, mathematical modelling, and epidemiological theory suggest that we can expect more societal benefit from isolation and quarantine in Phases 4 and 5. We don't know whether this will prove to be true, because these measures have never been widely applied in these phases. There's good reason to believe that they will deliver benefits, but we can't be sure. One suggestion that has been made is that we should perform scientific trials to assess these measures with seasonal influenza, which we believe shares many characteristics with pandemic influenza. This may give us a better scientific case for taking these steps.

In the absence of absolute scientific justification, we must look toward expert advice and judgment, do what is fair to the people involved, and take actions that correspond in a reasonable way to the expected benefits for society. This approach is no different than that of many decisions in everyday life outside of a pandemic. In the individual medical care of people, and even in making societal decisions, we often don't have absolute scientific evidence. As the pandemic progresses, stronger scientific evidence may emerge as different parts of the world try to address their pandemic problems and collect data on their successes and failures.

RIGHTS AND RESPONSIBILITIES OF
HEALTH CARE WORKERS

What obligations do health care workers have to provide health care if doing so increases their own risk of developing influenza?

Health care workers who take care of people with influenza may have a higher risk of contracting influenza, of giving it to family and friends, and of dying. In affluent countries, we plan to implement all necessary precautions to reduce the risk that health care workers face. Despite this effort, delivering health care to someone with influenza is a form of close contact that will increase personal risk.

Some argue that health care workers are not obliged to undertake the unusual risks posed by a pandemic. Others propose that health professionals should pursue their duties to society with personal safety as a secondary concern, much as police or firefighters sometimes put themselves in harm's way. During the SARS outbreak in 2003, a large number of health care workers worldwide became ill in the course of their work, and some died. Most health care workers in Toronto and elsewhere showed their commitment in the face of danger, but some refused to care for people with SARS. A small number were dismissed for failure to report for work. Following SARS, many health care workers questioned the adequacy of the protection they had been offered.

Dr. Lam's Perspective
Working During a Pandemic
Like many health care professionals, I believe that caring for sick people is a calling, and not simply a job. Not turning up at the hospital during a pandemic would not only jeopardize my career and my colleagues, it would endanger the well-being of the public, who rely on Canada's doctors, nurses, and allied health professionals.

I am also a husband and a father. Just as I believe that the Canadian public has a right to make a claim upon my skills and services, especially in a time of crisis, I believe that my son has a legitimate expectation that his father will be around for a while. My wife is also a physician. My son certainly can make a claim that he should not be orphaned, which is at least as legitimate as the public's right to receive medical services. My colleagues have family members whom they love dearly, and some of the bitterest lingering memories from SARS are those of health care professionals who did not feel they or their families were adequately protected or helped during a time of crisis.

Of course, going to work in a hospital during an influenza pandemic is not the same thing as standing in front of a firing squad. It's probably more comparable to entering a minefield. I wouldn't do it unless I had a good reason to do so—for instance, if I happened to be a sapper whose job was to clear the mines so that others wouldn't wander into the fields and be killed. I would undertake to demine a field only with the right equipment and a clear idea of how to go about my task. On most days, most sappers go home after successfully clearing a number of mines. Nonetheless, sometimes sappers get blown up, and sometimes health care workers who care for people with infectious diseases catch those illnesses.

Unlike soldiers, health care workers are private citizens, and though I plan to take care of patients in the event of a pandemic, it's not my place to judge any of my colleagues who decide to do otherwise. I certainly plan to take every possible measure to ensure that I'm around to see my son grow up. In a war, a minority of soldiers are actually at the front engaged in combat. A larger number play a supporting role, ferrying supplies, caring for the wounded, and stepping up to the front if needed. During an influenza pandemic, face-to-face health care will be the front line. Just as a soldier in battle should reasonably expect that the rest of the army will bring up the rear, a health care professional should be able to expect the moral as well as material support of society during the next pandemic.

The ethical conflict that health care workers face during a pandemic is not only the conflict between their individual and legal rights to health and safety under our occupational health legislation, and their professional obligation to help the sick. It is also a conflict between their duties to society and their obligations to the people in their own lives. Health care workers must weigh the risk that they may bring harm to family members and friends by possibly infecting them with influenza, as well as the duty that they have of being available to care for their family members if they fall ill. They must consider the risk of not being able to fulfill commitments such as raising children, being a spouse, and completing other important personal obligations, if they become seriously ill or die.

The argument that health care workers have an increased obligation to provide care notes that health care workers have freely chosen their profession along with its attendant risks; that because they have more ability to help than most members of society, they have a correspondingly greater responsibility to help; and that there is an implicit social contract that expects health care workers to be available in times of emergency.

Professional bodies representing nurses, physicians, and other health care professionals should consider these issues and provide clear statements to guide the conduct of their members during a pandemic. The process by which health care workers' obligations during a pandemic are defined must include the input of front-line workers and must be open in its goals and principles. The result of this process must set expectations that are reasonable, must be fair in the distribution of risk among health care workers, and must include a mechanism through which criticisms can be voiced. This discourse should occur before a pandemic, but it may need to be revisited both before and during a pandemic.

People's individual situations are quite variable, both in their potential importance in pandemic health care and in their personal responsibilities. We suggest that during a pandemic, health care workers must examine the conflicting risks and obligations in their lives and make individual decisions about whether to work, while being mindful of what their profession expects of them.

If necessary, the Canadian Emergencies Act does make it legally possible to compel health care workers to deliver health care, with refusal punishable by imprisonment and substantial fines. At the time of writing, Ontario is in the process of passing Bill 56, which would give its government broader powers during an emergency. The bill's language suggests the power to compel persons to work in an emergency situation; it would give officials the power to implement measures as they deem necessary "in order to prevent, respond to or alleviate the effects of the emergency."[6] People who refuse to comply could be fined $100,000 and imprisoned for one year. "This is very dangerous . . . If we were in the military, I would have no objections to . . . working under conditions that may not be of my choosing.

But I am a private individual. I am not part of a military service,"[1] said Dr. Merrilee Fullerton, an Ottawa family physician.

The Ontario Medical Association is opposed to any suggestion of forced work by physicians and other professionals, and at the time of this writing it is seeking assurances from the Ontario government regarding the rights and safety of its members and their families in the event of a pandemic. The association asks that there be assurances of adequate protective equipment when delivering health care, consideration of danger pay during a pandemic, and government-supplied life insurance for those professionals who succumb to influenza illness.

Dr. Ross Upshur, associate professor at the University of Toronto's Joint Centre for Bioethics, has said, "My own opinion is that legislation is a very draconian way of going about it that will likely not do anything but alienate and enrage physicians."[7] In the United States, a federally declared state of emergency gives the U.S. government enhanced powers to compel people to work. Forced work is a very ethically and practically undesirable option. It interferes with people's freedom of choice in a way that exposes them to the risk of physical harm. Health care is a complex professional task that requires commitment and motivation to be performed well. A health care worker who is forced to work is not likely to perform well, and during a pandemic may even make matters worse for his or her patients and co-workers.

It is reasonable that if health care workers are willing to put themselves in harm's way for the benefit of society, society has some corresponding obligations to them. Health care workers should be given appropriate protection from infection at work, and the health of their families should be considered. Such protection might mean prioritizing health care workers to receive antiviral medications for preventive treatment, or being the first recipients of a vaccine once it is available. It is reasonable to ask that governments should compensate health care workers for the dangers they expose themselves to in the course of their duties, provide financial support for those health care workers who become ill and unable to work while caring for influenza patients, and provide life insurance in the case of their demise.

WHO WILL GET SCARCE RESOURCES?

How will we prioritize the use of resources, such as limited supplies of medical equipment, medications, or vaccines, during a pandemic?

Rationing

We may have to acknowledge that rationing of scarce resources is necessary. We must turn to scientific evidence, societal values, and priorities for guidance.

If the influenza pandemic is as serious as some predict, during Phase 6 there may be a sudden surge in demand for medical services in all countries. The majority of people can be expected to recover without needing much medical treatment, but some will require professional help and even hospitalization and intensive care measures. Since a large number of people may develop influenza during a pandemic, even if the proportion of these people who require professional medical care is small, they may still represent a very large addition to the usual numbers of people seeking medical care. This demand may overwhelm medical care systems, creating shortages of medications, medical equipment, and health care workers. If this situation arises, who gets first access to these limited resources?

Health Care Rationing

We ration health care during non-pandemic times. This process is an accepted practice in the ethical landscape of our medical system. For example, people in Canada do not go directly to see a specialist. They see their family doctor, who decides how to care for them, and who also makes a decision whether their problem requires the care of a specialist. When new vaccinations are developed, different jurisdictions decide whether to make these vaccinations available free of charge to the public, or to require people to pay for them. If someone needs a specialized test like an MRI scan, there is usually a waiting period. However, if someone has an urgent health problem requiring that test, the wait is shorter.

All these are forms of rationing medical care. They balance society's obligations to pay for certain types of care against the legitimacy and urgency of people's needs. Most Canadians believe that our medical care system, although it may not be perfect, embodies principles of fairness and society's obligations to care for individual people who are ill. Meanwhile, we are a wealthy country. When people in Canada really need some kind of medical care, they can usually get it. The difference during a pandemic is that needs may significantly exceed the supply of resources, requiring more strict rationing during a difficult time.

Here is a hypothetical situation: If, during Phase 6 of a pandemic, there are only five breathing machines (ventilators) in a hospital, and that hospital has 15 people who will otherwise die unless they are placed on a ventilator, a rather awful decision must be made. This ethical dilemma pits individuals against one another in their legitimate needs and expectations of medical care. All human beings have a right to medical care in proportion to their needs. However, if the resources do not exist to provide care for everyone, who will get those limited resources? How will this be decided?

The reality is that accepting certain values and priorities changes the order in which people receive scarce resources. In choosing which five people to put on the ventilators, there are no absolute moral guidelines. If we prioritize maximizing the effectiveness of medical treatments, we must turn to scientific evidence if it predicts that one patient with certain illness features will probably do better than another patient with different features of illness. This evidence may favour giving the ventilator to a "less sick" person who needs a ventilator instead of another person who also needs it, if the "less sick" person has a greater chance of surviving through treatment. If we prioritize saving the largest number of potential life years (the remaining number of years that a person is expected to live), this judgment favours giving the ventilators to children and young adults ahead of elderly people. If we wish to avoid making children orphans, this priority favours putting parents on ventilators if they need them. If we prioritize maintaining essential societal services, then health care workers, fire and police workers, and utility workers would be put on ventilators ahead of other people if they become critically ill. When everyone's legitimate claims to health care cannot be met at once, the ethical dilemma of who gets medical care first must be informed partly by science, and partly by societal values and priorities.

The ventilator dilemma is an extreme one, chosen to illustrate a point, and one that few people will ever need to confront. More people may be affected by the ethical conflict in distributing scarce supplies of antiviral medications and vaccines. Other aspects of antivirals and vaccines have been addressed in previous chapters. The ethical dilemma is that many people may make a claim upon medications and vaccines, possibly in excess of the available resources. Priority groups will need to be established. Things will not play themselves out quite as starkly as in our ventilator example, because the risks of not receiving a medication or vaccine are not categorically fatal. Nonetheless, the core nature of this conflict is the same.

Scientific knowledge rarely gives us clear answers. Instead, it often highlights difficult choices that societies need to make. For example, children over age two have among the best odds of surviving seasonal influenza without any treatment. As a consequence, in many countries' current pandemic plans normally healthy children over age two have lower priority to receive antiviral medications and vaccines. Can we accept this, as a society? Not every child over age two who develops influenza will survive, but it may be that more are destined to survive with no treatment than people in some other age groups. Young adults died in greater proportions in past pandemics than is their norm during seasonal influenza. Do we put their treatment before that of young children? Or do we believe that children have a right to priority care simply because they are children, and thus should receive scarce medications ahead of young adults, even if most will survive without the medications? This is one of the many dilemmas that has put any sort of priority list in question.

Individual Rights Versus Societal Benefit

There can be conflict between people's individual rights to obtain resources that may be helpful to them, and the obligations of governments to distribute scarce resources in a way that achieves the most societal benefit.

Current controversies about the stockpiling of Tamiflu are an example of this ethical dilemma. In many countries, individuals have tried to obtain personal stockpiles of this medication, which is expected to have some usefulness in addressing a pandemic strain of influenza. This has led to a worldwide "shortage" of the drug. In many places Roche, the manufacturer of the drug, temporarily suspended the public sale of this medication, with priority sales going to government and institutional pandemic stockpiling and addressing current seasonal influenza outbreaks. We have outlined elsewhere our view that this is a temporary problem.

Ethically, however, while this "shortage" exists, it gives us conflicts between people's individual rights to try to help themselves, and governments' responsibility to ensure that scarce resources are used to achieve the maximum amount of good for society. The claim could be made that anyone has the right to personally stockpile Tamiflu in case it will be helpful to her. However, there is an ethical conflict if this drug is in short supply, and if government is able to use it to achieve a greater good for society than a number of people with individual supplies. Is it a wise use of resources for one person to have a stock of Tamiflu that she may never need to use, while someone else who needs it receives none because of its scarcity?

Another ethical conflict arises from the possibility that the inappropriate use of Tamiflu by individuals—underdosing, inconsistent dosing, or using it in the wrong situation—may promote antiviral resistance. If this occurs, people who are subsequently infected with a resistant strain will discover that Tamiflu is less effective or ineffective in helping them. In this case, an individual acting upon his own right to try to help himself may have a negative impact on the health of others in society, thus interfering with other people's rights to health. If antiviral resistance is created by individuals' inappropriate use of a medication, it also interferes with governments' ability to fulfill their task of deploying scarce resources in a way that helps people.

Tamiflu delivers impressive results in preventing seasonal influenza illness.[8] The science is less impressive in its effectiveness at actually treating illness. During a pandemic, Tamiflu or other medications may have a similar profile: very useful in prevention but less successful in treatment. If there is a limited supply of antivirals, how much should be used for treatment and how much for preventive treatment? Might governments decide that their responsibility to wisely use a scarce resource in order to maximize societal benefit means prioritizing the use of this drug to prevent illness, as a higher priority than treating it? Such a decision would mean giving the drug to people who are not sick ahead of those who are sick.

We feel that at present, governments and pharmaceutical companies are taking the right approach in creating national stockpiles and prioritizing sales of antiviral medications to governments and health care institutions. Our support assumes a commitment on the part of governments and medical institutions to use stockpiles of antiviral medications wisely in defence of the public interest.

Making Resource Decisions

All segments of society should have a say in how scarce resources are distributed, and should be able to see in an open and honest way how decisions are made.

Governments and decision-makers should make clear the values and beliefs that underpin their choices of certain priorities. Before a pandemic, the priority-setting process should include the input of the public. During a pandemic, there may be insufficient time for full public consultation on urgent questions, but public input should be sought if possible. Decisions made without direct public consultation should be grounded in values that are believed to be commonly held. They should be openly communicated and made with a profound commitment to using scarce resources to achieve the greatest societal good.

If there is a time when not everyone can receive the resources to which they make a claim, it is fair that all segments of society should at least have the opportunity to clearly see and examine the reasons for governments' and institutions' decisions. Not everyone will agree upon decisions that are made. There should be room to constructively criticize and re-examine issues as a pandemic progresses.

GLOBAL PERSPECTIVES

Global priorities may not be identical to local ones.

Currently the WHO is urging all countries to create pandemic plans, as well as robust surveillance networks for animal and human health. The value of these networks in the response and management of a pandemic is unquestionable. The efficient operation of these surveillance networks is necessary if we are to have any possibility of delaying or averting a pandemic in Phase 4 or 5.

One ethical problem that arises is that many of the countries that are asked to create or strengthen influenza surveillance networks, and that arguably have the most work to do in this regard, are poor. In affluent countries, we debate whether to stockpile Tamiflu at $5 per dose. Meanwhile, $5 is higher than the annual health care budget available for some people living in sub-Saharan Africa. Many have limited resources and struggle with basic issues of food, water, sanitation, shelter, control of childhood diseases, HIV prevention, and other health challenges whose management we take for granted in affluent countries. If the limited resources of these countries are used for pandemic preparedness, this effort benefits both themselves and the rest of the world. However, if the majority of the cost is borne by the poor and vulnerable citizens of these countries, these limited resources are no longer available to undertake other important health activities. Pandemic preparedness addresses a real risk to human health whose timing is unpredictable, meanwhile many of the other health issues confronted by less affluent countries involve preventable causes of illness and death that have a steady, ongoing human toll. For instance, in Africa, malaria is the number one killer of children, particularly those

Eggs or Influenza?

Imagine asking a subsistence farmer in an H5N1-affected country who has a few chickens in his backyard whether he'd rather keep the chickens and eggs that provide his children with an important part of their diet, or kill them in order to address a real but hard to quantify risk of an influenza pandemic. Assume that the farmer has a full understanding of all the issues in this book, including the possibility of the chickens becoming ill and even infecting his children. Despite this knowledge, the farmer might still decide to keep the chickens. In the immediate future, his children being hungry could be a concrete outcome of losing the chickens, while the timing and genesis of an influenza pandemic are still topics of scientific debate. The farmer might also decide that his children's right to have an adequate diet, including protein from poultry, might outweigh the potential risks posed to them by the chickens. The farmer might correctly point out that there seems to be a tension between his children's right to be properly fed and the world's claim upon animal health surveillance and control systems.

under five years of age. A child dies of malaria every 30 seconds.[9] There is an ethical conflict if poor countries are asked to do things that benefit the entire world, but at the cost of the basic needs of their own citizens.

Elsewhere, we have discussed animal health. Animal culls are estimated to have affected 300 million largely poor farmers at this point, at a cost of US$10 billion. The benefits of controlling the spread of H5N1 in domestic poultry accrue to the entire world. The costs are borne by farmers and individual governments, but compensation is not universally adequate or equal. Domestic poultry are often an important source of cash and dietary protein. It is only fair that farmers should be compensated for their losses by everyone else in the world who benefits from these culls. Less affluent countries may reasonably ask that more affluent countries, who benefit equally in pandemic risk reduction from animal control measures, contribute financially to mitigate these losses.

When we reach Phases 4 and 5 of the pandemic, one of the responsibilities of the WHO will be to make travel recommendations. They may include border measures and the recommendation that people avoid non-essential travel to certain regions. SARS showed us how regions, such as Toronto, that were placed under travel advisories suffered serious economic losses. In 2003, the overall estimated economic losses from SARS were just under $1 billion for Toronto and $40 billion worldwide.[10-11] Travel measures implemented in Phases 4 and 5 may avert a pandemic. If this happens, regions that have been economically and societally affected by travel measures will have suffered losses in the interest of protecting the rest of the world.

World health authorities and individual nations, especially affluent ones, must recognize that border measures taken on one side of the world may have the greatest benefit for people on the other side of the world, with the costs naturally falling to the place where the actions are taken. Material and financial support should be made available to people who are willing to make these sacrifices. A commitment to this kind of global solidarity will make it more possible for individual countries to take appropriate actions even if there are associated local costs.

CHAPTER 14

PRACTICAL PROBLEMS OF AN INFLUENZA PANDEMIC

THIS CHAPTER IN ONE PAGE . . .

• A pandemic may be a threatening experience, and a legitimate human reaction to threat is fear. Do not be ruled by fear, but try to understand what is happening around you during a pandemic, and make decisions based upon the things that are important in your life.

• The next influenza pandemic will provide many practical challenges in all industries and businesses. The economic impact may be significant.

• Because of the increased demand on health care, medical care will be delivered in novel ways that may involve health care professionals and others performing roles that are different from their normal ones.

• Crucial public health measures may change over time.

• An influenza pandemic is a no-win situation for politicians.

"The fear in the hearts of people just withered them. They were afraid to go out, afraid to do anything . . . You just lived from day to day, did what you had to do and not think about the future. If you asked a neighbor for help, they wouldn't do so because they weren't taking any chances . . . Even if there was war, the war was removed from us, you know—on the other side . . . This malignancy . . . it was right at our very doors."

—Susanna Turner, Philadelphia hospital
volunteer during the 1918–19 pandemic[1]

"It took away all your community life, you had no school life, you had no church life, you had nothing . . . People were afraid to kiss one another, to eat with one another, to have anything that made contact because that's how you got the flu. It destroyed these contacts and destroyed the intimacy amongst people."

—William Sardo, Washington, D.C., resident
during the 1918–19 pandemic[1]

FEAR

Some may argue that a prevailing "culture of fear" heightens our sense of vulnerability to murky, unpredictable dangers. They might suggest that there's not much point in feeling overly afraid of an influenza pandemic before there is one. We tend to agree. However, taking reasonable precautions against a danger and making preparations to avert or mitigate it should not be equated with "feeling afraid." We all wear seatbelts, although most of us are not actively fearful of crashing every time we travel in a car.

There are facts that no one will be able to change during a pandemic: for example, the ways in which a virus spreads, and the degree to which it causes serious illness and death. Thankfully, we know a great deal about influenza, and we can already begin to plan both the public health and personal measures that may help mitigate its damage. We know influenza spreads in droplets. We know it's useful to wash your hands. We know that most people who develop influenza recover, but more people than usual die during pandemics.

The individual reactions to an actual, current threat are a somewhat different issue. A reasonable person would feel afraid if the brakes were to fail in her car. A reasonable person, upon hearing that a new strain of influenza to which no one in the world has immunity had just ignited, rapidly spreading clusters of disease, would be concerned that he or his loved ones could be affected by this virus. It is normal to be afraid in the face of a real threat. During a pandemic, we encourage you to look past your fear, and decide what the situation means to you.

Your experience of an influenza pandemic may be governed as much by your human reactions to a pandemic as by the events around you. If you do not become ill from influenza, you might still experience anxiety, a sense of mistrust toward those around you, and a sense of personal vulnerability. If you become ill, you may be afraid of your illness, you may experience stigmatization and isolation, and you may even have a sense of helplessness. If these emotions become part of your experience of an influenza pandemic, acknowledge that this is the case and figure out how to move forward. Review what you know about the facts of influenza. Find out what your local public health agency advises. From this information, make practical decisions about the things that you can control in your own life in order to minimize your chances of being negatively affected by the pandemic. Figure out which facts of your situation you can affect, whether that means changing the way you travel to work so that you're not in crowds or preparing food for a neighbour who has become ill.

During a pandemic, decide how much attention you want to pay to international news. Once a pandemic is fully under way, it may be that the most important issues in your life are very practical local issues, and your most relevant day-to-day public health advice comes from professionals in your city, town, or province. The overall management of an influenza pandemic by public health and medical workers absolutely must take a broad, international perspective. Whether you, personally, need to check the WHO website twice daily for updates on the international events of the pandemic is a matter of personal choice. Some people will feel that they gain a greater sense of perspective and control by closely watching what happens around the world. Others may prefer to check the international news only occasionally and may decide to focus their attention more on local issues and advice, which have more practical relevance for them.

Continue to do things that give meaning and shape to your life. Read, write, exercise, be in touch with friends and family—even if only by telephone. Take pleasure in small things. As much as you do to keep physically well, do an equal amount to stay mentally healthy.

IMPACTS ON INDUSTRIES AND BUSINESSES

All industries and businesses may be affected by an influenza pandemic, and each will face its own varied difficulties. All industries may face disruptions to their workforces: a number of workers will be ill at some point, some will stay at home out of fear initially, some will need to stay at home to take care of ill family members, the closure of schools may keep workers at home to care for children, isolation and quarantine would remove people from the workforce for a few days each, and community containment measures such as "snow days" would have significant impacts. The many unknowns associated with an influenza pandemic mean that we cannot prepare for every possible problem.

Canadian Manufacturers and Exporters, an industry lobby group, projects that an influenza pandemic could cost the Canadian economy $60 billion. The American pandemic plan estimates that health costs in the United States, not accounting for economic disruption, would be US$181 billion for a moderate pandemic. McKibbin and Sidorenko, analysts for the Lowy Institute for International Policy, explore a variety of scenarios ranging from a mild outbreak, which would result in a US$330 billion loss in global economic output, to an "ultra" pandemic, which would entail a US$4.4 trillion loss in global economic output.[2]

In economic terms, the principal impacts of a pandemic are not likely to come from deaths. Rather, they will come from illness and its associated treatment costs, employee absenteeism, disruptions to economic production and trade, and changes in consumer preferences and consumption. Perfectly healthy people will make different consumer choices and conduct their lives differently during a pandemic, resulting in an economic impact even if they never become ill. Travel and tourism will be hurt. Hospitality, entertainment, and consumer spending will be affected as people spend less time in busy public venues. Industries that rely on international trade may be hampered by international border restrictions. Economic disruption may have a domino effect: the reduced ability of a few key types of businesses to operate may cause widespread negative effects in other businesses. Schools and educational institutions may see their activities limited or halted temporarily by illness and public health measures, possibly creating child-care problems, which may further increase employee absenteeism. In short, a serious Phase 6 pandemic has the potential to create practical problems for everyone in society, not all of which are predictable.

Dr. Lam's Perspective: SARS from Behind the Mask, *National Post*, April 19, 2003

I never knew how much I relied upon lip-reading in my job as an emergency physician until I became unable to see the faces of my patients. For the past two weeks, going to work in a SARS-protected environment has meant spending hours smothered in an N95 mask, wrapped in an isolation gown, wearing eye protection and gloves. Patients in the emergency department are masked as well, so we peer at each other like disembodied eyes and hairstyles. Suddenly, I cannot understand what anyone is saying. Words are usually obscured by accents and the noise of the emergency department, but now they are also muffled by the mask material itself, and I cannot watch people's lips. I now realize how much I need to see the movement of lips to understand speech.

"I see berry berry vizzy," says my patient.

"What?" I say.

"I see fizzy," says my patient.

"You feel dizzy?" I say.

My patient nods, finally.

Already, SARS is becoming a "new normal" for those of us who continue to work in Toronto hospitals. Many hospital clinics are closed, but for those of us who remain in what are deemed to be essential services, we are becoming accustomed to lining up in a tent in the back of the hospital in order to get into work. All the entrances are sealed except the emergency entrance, where patients pass through a parked bus borrowed from the public transit system to be screened, and the back entrance, where staff are processed in the tent. There our temperatures are taken as we file past infection control workers with thermometers. We answer daily questionnaires about our physical condition, whether we have worked at other hospitals, whether we have travelled, and whether we have cared for SARS patients. If we are deemed to be "clean," we are issued our daily gown and mask, which we must don in order to enter the hospital. Each day there seem to be different models of masks, and staff members are developing individual preferences regarding them. All of them are smothering and hot. One of the nurses in the emergency department brought smiley stickers, which could be scratched and sniffed to release a strawberry scent. On that day, we had strawberry smiley stickers on the exhalation ports of the N95 masks.

One of my fellow physicians refused to have a sticker on his mask, saying, "There's nothing funny about this."

He's right, of course. It's not funny, and we're all scared.

During normal times, the emergency department

carries a sense of rough-and-ready fatalism. Bad things happen, and disaster wheels in, sirens blaring. We jump into the fray, try to save a life, and then the next patient rolls in. Now we feel that the danger of SARS lurks in our midst, and, more than just responding to it, we may become its victims. Many of the SARS cases in Toronto have been among health care workers. Even though SARS patients are isolated from the public, we must continue to care for them. For us, it is not far away. We are comforted by the fact that SARS cases in health care workers occurred only, it seems, before current infection control measures were undertaken.

It is the unknown that is most sinister. At present, laboratories around the world spend sleepless night trying to isolate the SARS pathogen. The mode of transmission is unclear but our main line of defence, quarantine and isolation, is an effort to break transmission. So we are fighting an enemy that we cannot see with weapons of unknown effect. What we grasp are the screening questionnaires and treatment protocols that outline who should be suspected of SARS, who should be isolated, who should have the myriad swabs and tests drawn, who should be admitted to hospital, and who should simply be reassured that, as far as we can tell, they do not have SARS.

The protocols have been changing. Before leaving for each shift at the hospital, I check my email to learn if the guidelines are different today. I print out the flow charts, to see if all the little arrows go to the same boxes they led to on the last flow chart. Patients whom we would have sent home in the first days of the outbreak are now being admitted to hospital. It is normal for things to change in medicine, for dogma to be contradicted by a new finding, and for a new way of treatment to render another incorrect. However, this usually happens over years, and we have time to nurse our old folly and coddle our new wisdom. Now, with our knowledge of SARS changing daily, we have no time to lull ourselves into any illusion of understanding. The staff in the emergency department all follow the daily number of cases, the number of fatalities. It is like watching flood water rise at a dike and wondering if it will overflow.

I and a fellow physician were deciding how to manage a patient who was struggling to breathe. We decided to isolate the patient and treat him as a suspected SARS case even though he did not meet the criteria in the flow chart of that day. Why did we do this? The situation of this patient who was struggling to breathe didn't quite make sense. It just "didn't look right" to our clinical instinct, that sacred gut reaction of medicine. My colleague said, "If we don't isolate him now, we may look back and think we were idiots."

What he meant is that if we missed one case because it didn't fit the guidelines, the potential consequences could be immense. Days after, the protocol was altered to accommodate the consideration of SARS in patients such as this who presented with apparently other respiratory problems in an "atypical manner." As a profession, we're still figuring it out.

In the lounge, there is mostly quiet, and the little talk is about SARS. At breaks, everyone drinks water. The masks cause a very dry mouth—it's like working in a hot fog. One of the nurses said one night, "If I thought that by coming to work I could catch something that could kill me, I wouldn't come to work."

This thought has crossed many of our minds, of

course. We hope that none of us will contract SARS or die from it, and I know of no one who has stopped coming to work out of fear. I keep on thinking that this is what health care has always been like, that in the past few decades we in North America have been briefly sheltered from humanity's long history of plagues, epidemics, and deadly scourges. It makes me think that maybe we've had a bit of a honeymoon, that perhaps now we're getting a little taste of the real marriage between humanity and infectious disease.

Early in the outbreak, I advised a woman that she would need to be admitted to hospital for emergency surgery to treat a life-threatening problem. She agreed but asked me anxiously, "Tell me the truth, do you have SARS in this hospital?"

At that time, my answer was that we did not. The patient was very relieved, despite her other medical problems. Now my answer would be different. We now have SARS patients who have come through our emergency department and are admitted to our hospital. For the moment, our clinics remain closed, and in the emergency department we try to be vigilant for SARS, care for all of our patients through our mask and gown barriers, and protect ourselves.

The masks, in addition to making it difficult to understand speech, impair much other communication. My conversations with patients seem distant and impoverished when I cannot see a grimace or the understanding of a grin. These expressions contain many unspoken clues to diagnosis, as well as a sense of a person's human situation. My patients seem in danger of becoming random garbled speech emanating from a blue mask perched on top of a body. I must seem equally surreal, as a doctor floating through the room in my gown, waving my white-gloved hands. I find myself gesturing more, using a sort of mime to transmit the meanings that are usually visible on my face.

For the moment, we in the hospitals continue to watch the flood of new cases, of daily news reports, and of the strange changes in our workplace getting close to the top of our dike. We hope that this flood will not overflow into the community around us. It is a pleasurable freedom to leave work, to be able to breathe, to sit in a restaurant and understand what people are talking about. The numbers of new SARS cases seem to be decreasing. It's too early to say what will happen, but hopefully it will burn itself out and leave us with a new appreciation of being able to see one another's faces. If not, we will continue to learn about SARS and about ourselves.

MEDICAL CARE IN A PANDEMIC

Even without a pandemic, medical care systems in many countries are stretched trying to meet the demands for regular services. During a pandemic, systems may have to change the ways that they operate in order to give more care to a greater number of people. In addition to a sudden increase in the need for services, during Phase 6 there may be fewer health care workers available. Some could be sick or dead, some may be at home caring for their families; hopefully only small numbers would refuse to work. Those who continue to work will see their working speed reduced by the increased emphasis upon infection control practices. While pandemic needs are addressed, other health needs will continue and cannot be ignored during the months and years of a pandemic. Broken bones will still have to be set. Babies will still be born.

Medical care may operate differently and may require the use of non-standard care providers. People may need to work in different roles within the system, and there may be a need to rapidly train new workers and volunteers. If elective surgeries are cancelled, operating room nurses may be asked to take care of influenza patients. Health care students, dentists, veterinarians, and others may all be asked to do things like start intravenous lines or administer immunizations. People who have never worked in health care may be employed, or may volunteer, to do things like feeding and cleaning sick people. There will be great advantages to delivering medical information and advice by telephone and Internet, requiring fewer resources and reducing the potential for the spread of influenza.

Increasing the availability of medical care but ensuring a crucial level of quality and accountability may be a challenge. Having less-experienced people perform certain tasks would mean that more mistakes are possible. Telephone medical advice may be delivered at a level of complexity that in non-pandemic times we would never consider without in-person medical assessment, creating more possibilities for error in the advice given and the way advice is understood. It may be necessary to decide whether a reduction in the quality of a particular service is justified by an increased availability of that service. More people can get advice if a nurse or doctor gives it on the phone. More people may receive medical care if 20 students and volunteers are available to deliver care instead of one fully qualified and trained professional.

The public may have to accept that unusual circumstances create different professional standards and change the parameters of medical liability. This concept already exists during non-pandemic times. A family doctor in downtown Toronto would not consider performing neurosurgery, because a nearby neurosurgeon could take better care of a patient needing such surgery. But on rare occasions, non-neurosurgeon physicians in remote parts of Canada have performed life-saving neurosurgery, when evacuation services were unable to bring a patient to a neurosurgeon in a timely manner. This is professionally and ethically justifiable, because in a particular circumstance it is sometimes the best option for that particular patient.

During a pandemic, professionals still have responsibilities and should be held accountable for their actions. However, dermatologists who care for critically ill influenza patients should not be held to the professional standards of a respirologist or lung specialist during a non-pandemic period. Rather, the care that they are expected to deliver is that of a non-respirologist physician, acting in the best interest of patients during extreme circumstances. If telephone advice is given in good faith as the best professional advice possible, but the patient dies, that telephone advice cannot be held to the same standard as advice given after a physician has performed a full in-person physical assessment. If volunteers are manning ambulances, they would need to receive enough basic training so that their actions are both useful and accountable, but they could not be expected to engage in all the complex tasks that a fully trained paramedic would be able to undertake. Medical systems will need to be aware of their responsibility to constantly re-evaluate the situation, to be flexible yet coordinated, in order to ensure that the kind of care that is being delivered is the best possible at that point in time.

Infection prevention and control systems are usually simple in conception but filled with practical problems, which we personally had ample experience with in Toronto during the 2003 outbreak of SARS. Where should someone who is coughing sit while waiting to see a nurse or doctor? Where and when should a person's temperature be taken? If care providers are to wash their hands between all patient encounters, what if the only sinks available close by are inside the potentially contaminated patient rooms?

In most Canadian hospitals, answering these questions has required a culture change among health care providers in regard to infection control practices. These adaptations are an often challenging process in which health care providers have had to change the very way they perform key, routine parts of their job to accommodate the use of masks, gloves, goggles, gowns, and other infection control measures. There has been a need to construct new isolation rooms, install new ventilation equipment, and adjust supply chains for infection control supplies. Much of this shift began during the SARS outbreak, and it continues to be refined. There are large capital costs and logistical challenges associated with redesign and reconstruction of hospital patient rooms and departments.

Phase 6 of an influenza pandemic may create logistical dilemmas for medical care systems that are large in scale and previously unimaginable. No medical care system will be able to either completely anticipate or prepare for the practical problems created by an actual pandemic, because this event is unpredictable in timing, severity, dynamics, and magnitude.

THE "RIGHT" PUBLIC HEALTH MEASURES
WILL CHANGE OVER TIME

The public health interventions in Phases 4, 5, and 6 of a pandemic are implemented on a "to the best of our knowledge" basis. Actions require careful consideration and reasoning, but there is scientific uncertainty surrounding the exact impact of public health interventions upon influenza pandemics. Pandemics just haven't happened often and recently enough to provide the data to build a scientifically leakproof case for public health measures.

Some specific decisions about what to do and when to do it cannot be made in advance, because they will be closely linked to the virus's characteristics as well as to the way each phase plays out. Relevant variables that cannot be known at present include the virus's virulence (its tendency to cause serious illness and kill people), the attack rate in different age groups, and how much resistance develops to antiviral drugs. We have plausible predictions of some characteristics such as the duration of asymptomatic viral shedding, the duration of infectiousness before and after the onset of symptoms, and the expected large-droplet nature of influenza transmission, from our general knowledge of influenza. For example, if the attack rate is very high in children, or children are a major channel for infecting adults, a relevant public health action would be to consider closing schools. If children are rarely infected by the pandemic strain, then this measure would not be useful.

The application of current public health and medical knowledge of influenza is both valuable and essential. The science of influenza is also growing at an unprecedented rate. There are historical data from previous pandemics, there is sophisticated mathematical modelling, and there is a wealth of clinical knowledge about how to treat individual sick people and control infection. These will inform actions during a pandemic, but nonetheless these actions will need to be constantly evaluated and modified as the pandemic progresses. When governments and public health bodies intervene in a pandemic, they will simultaneously try to learn what works. The choice of action is also very dependent upon the pandemic phase. Public health actions are expected to change as a pandemic progresses, and changes should not be viewed as evidence of a lack of knowledge or consistency on the part of governments and public health authorities. The reality of changing public health actions through the course of a pandemic is an expected feature of an intelligent, well-informed, strategic response to pandemic influenza.

Some decisions may prove to have been wrong but will have been the best possible decisions given the knowledge that existed at the time they were made. Others will have been correct decisions but may lose their relevance in the face of a changing pandemic.

In Phases 4 and 5, we still believe, public health measures may have some chance of averting a pandemic. If they do not, then such actions would at least slow things down or limit damage. In Phase 6, experts believe, it is not possible to stop a pandemic, and the focus of public health action is to limit illness, death, and social disruption. Public health measures will disrupt people's lives and may limit their freedoms. It's a tough pill to swallow when people are asked to drastically disrupt their lives for a hard-to-define benefit.

We believe that the best way to maintain the public's trust and confidence in both government and institutions, as well as within society in general, is to be honest about these limitations. When public health measures are implemented, they will be essentially predicated upon the cooperation of the public, yet their exact benefit will be impossible to guarantee. This being the case, governments and institutions owe it to the public to explain the rationale behind public health decisions, and to be honest about what benefit can be expected. Despite everything, the pandemic may progress. Once Phase 6 comes, it will run its course. Hopefully, public health action and public cooperation with these measures will make things better than they otherwise would have been.

A NO-WIN SITUATION FOR POLITICIANS

In the politics of managing an influenza pandemic, the stakes are high and the parameters that inform decision-making are constantly changing. Decisions depend upon goals, but there can be a variety of legitimate and conflicting goals and the measures of success are difficult to determine. Phases 4 and 5 will bring many "no right answer" choices. When we reach a pandemic's Phase 6, it is likely that significant human, social, and economic losses can be expected, regardless of what political decisions are made.

Take the example of international border measures. They may create large economic disruptions. If stringent border measures are imposed in Phase 4 or 5, but a pandemic does not develop further and no pandemic cases cross a border, decision-makers may be criticized for taking "unnecessary" action and disrupting a nation's economy. On the other hand, if infection gets past a border despite travel measures, which will certainly happen if we get to Phase 6, decision-makers may be criticized either for imposing it unnecessarily because it was "unsuccessful" or for not imposing it strictly enough, so that it "failed." In fact, no such measure can "succeed" in any absolute way in Phase 6; its benefit could only be to delay widespread infection.

Decisions will be predicated upon social and political imperatives as well as upon science. There are trade-offs. Some decisions will be better for some goals and worse for others, and likewise some groups of people will be more satisfied with certain decisions than others. These tradeoffs may affect different groups of people in society unequally, and the stakes could be people's chances of surviving the pandemic.

The single most valuable thing to expect from a responsible government and functioning medical care system is well-informed and accountable information and decision-making. However, this may not seem like enough to people when their family members have become ill or died and they do not feel that everything possible was done to help them, or when people are afraid that they may become ill.

Countries are currently deciding upon preparations for an influenza pandemic, and this is in itself a politically perilous exercise. A government can spend a great deal of money to prepare for a pandemic, and if none arrives before the next election, it may be roundly criticized for overreacting to an overblown threat and wasting public money. Or a government can spend very little, and if its country is woefully unprepared at the onset of Phase 6 of a pandemic, it can expect to be held responsible for the illnesses of great numbers of people and the deaths of many.

Governments can be right, and governments can be wrong. Which is the case often depends on who is asking and who is being asked. Governments and citizens should both recognize the life cycle of influenza pandemics as one that spans decades and is influenced by events around the world. The natural pattern of this human health issue is to spend years in quiescence, then to occasionally and somewhat unpredictably make itself known, sometimes in dramatic fashion.

This life cycle is out of sync with most modern decision-making, which centres on the crisis of the moment and the issue of the day. This is why making decisions about a influenza pandemic is destined to be an exercise fraught with criticism. For leaders to make wise decisions, and for citizens to be able to evaluate and give feedback on those decisions, they must be viewed in the context of this long life cycle. Actions and preparations should be chosen to mitigate risk and enhance preparedness in ways that correspond with pandemic influenza being an ongoing risk to world human health. When we reach Phases 4, 5, and 6, it must be understood that regardless of what is done, each step into the next phase of an influenza pandemic will bring greater human and societal costs. The role of governments should be to try to minimize the negative effects that are otherwise expected. It is only if we have both honest, well-informed governments and responsible and cooperative societies that we can take meaningful action and have a chance of countering the forces of a global influenza pandemic.

CHAPTER 15

CONCLUSION

WHERE WE ARE

In Canada and around the world, debate continues in our media about the level of concern and preparedness appropriate to the possible threat of an influenza pandemic. It may be that we have been primed by the world experience of SARS. Certainly it is not the first time the world has been collectively worried about some source of threat to society. Y2K, terrorism, and other spectres have all recently had their turns in the scariness limelight.

The widespread discussion of a threat carries the subtext that "something bad will happen soon." In our popular culture of fast-paced film and televised wars, we have an implicit belief that once we've spotted the villain on-screen, within very short order he will commit a heinous crime. Astute observers will note, however, that fact does not necessarily pace its drama quite as well as fiction, and that whatever the predominant threat of the day, it may not immediately translate into the anticipated cataclysm. Not all threats materialize: the threatened computer meltdown of Y2K didn't occur. On the other hand, we can't dismiss all risks just because nothing bad has happened recently. Airliner hijackings were an issue of immense concern in the 1980s, we didn't hear much about them in the '90s, and we collectively forgot about them at the beginning of this millennium, until we were confronted with the events of 9/11.

As with on-screen drama, it would be nice to know where the story of bird flu ends. However, we can predict that it won't "end." To look overly hard for a clear conclusion to this story (such as a definitive statement on whether a pandemic will happen or not with a certain time frame) would be to miss an important lesson that emerges from our current knowledge of the phenomenon of influenza pandemics: they present a risk over time. There is a spectrum of risk, and the risk evolves in a way that has to do with the interplay among viral phenomena, animal health, and human health. An increase or decrease in media attention does not correlate well with the level of pandemic risk. If a pandemic does not materialize soon, then popular attention will likely dissipate.

Worldwide pandemics of some strain of influenza are recurring events in the cycle of human illness. They vary greatly in severity and impact, and their precise timing is unpredictable. The risk of H5N1 causing a pandemic is both a legitimate and a current threat. Our modern surveillance abilities and understanding of the evolution of pandemic risk give us a keen awareness of it. Some anticipate that H5N1 will cause a worldwide cataclysm. Others expect that not much of anything will come of H5N1. What science tells us with absolute clarity is that either of these scenarios could prove to be true, as could many intermediate possibilities. A different strain of influenza that is not currently attracting attention or has not yet even been discovered may end up causing our next pandemic years from now.

Our knowledge does give us a historically unprecedented opportunity to intervene. Some might ask, "If we don't know what's going to happen, how are we to decide what to do?" There's certainly no point trying to make absolute predictions about things that are inherently unpredictable. Instead, the key task is to consider the range of possible outcomes, and the paramount question becomes this: What are the reasonable things to do given that we understand the broad strokes of the issue, but that we do not know exactly what will happen?

In many areas of our lives, it would be nice to predict the future with certainty, whether choosing among personal health options or simply picking a route to take to work in the morning. Exact predictions often cannot be made, and we judge what may or may not happen in everyday choices. We may think that one route to work will not have a traffic jam, and then it does. We may take a medication to treat a problem, and it turns out to have unpleasant side effects. That's just the way it is. We tolerate some unknowns and ask ourselves to make reasonable decisions. This is the same challenge for the world's governments, public health organizations, and any individual person who would like to respond meaningfully to the risk of pandemic influenza in everyday life. The risk of pandemic influenza is unlikely to ever go away.

A health institution, public health organization, or government must realize that it is not worthwhile to redirect all its resources from all other activities toward pandemic preparedness, yet it would be irresponsible to make no plans whatsoever. The reasonable middle ground depends upon the resources available, the current state of knowledge, the science that emerges, social priorities, and the development of the current risk of a pandemic. Will tough decisions be made and subsequently criticized? Absolutely—this is our one guarantee. Criticism is a feature of an honest, functional society. It is useful for decision-makers as well as the public to understand in advance that things aren't going to work out perfectly.

A private individual should not build a hermetically sealed pandemic bunker but may consider keeping some extra food in the house and getting a flu shot. What about a personal stockpile of antiviral medications? On that question there is room for discussion, which will be most valuable if it is well-informed, level-headed, and based on a broad knowledge of principles and concepts, such as those we hope you have found in this book. The detailed, current information that we have included will change. The concepts will remain.

WHERE WE'RE GOING

The prospect of an influenza pandemic does present both a unique opportunity and a threat within our world society of the 21st century. The epidemics observed by Hippocrates, Livy, and Ebn-Al-Atir may have been influenza but were not pandemics. It may be that these episodes did not result in worldwide pandemics because people just didn't move around as much as they do today. Of course, these illnesses didn't get to North America—the ancient world didn't know that this continent existed. In contrast, in the 20th century, the emergence of three novel strains of influenza led on three occasions to pandemics. Each time, the whole world was involved. We may have our modern borders, but the ability of a kiss, a handshake, and a jumbo jet to spread influenza means that a new strain of influenza can span the globe in a time frame limited only by the speed of an airliner. SARS gave us a small, recent taste of that, but SARS was a faint shadow in comparison with the possible impact of a serious influenza pandemic.

The awareness of our global vulnerability affords the world an unprecedented collective opportunity. The potential for the spread of influenza transcends national boundaries. Local planning is crucial because a pandemic ultimately affects individual people in the places where they live. Nonetheless, agricultural, travel, and containment decisions made on one side of the globe may affect people thousands of kilometres away in a concrete and tangible way. Addressing pandemic risk in its current state and in its subsequent stages is of immensely greater value if undertaken with a spirit of global cooperation and an awareness of our interdependence. Whatever diplomatic conflicts we have, trade disputes we undergo, and wars we fight, an influenza pandemic is likely to affect us all. In World War I, the American troops spread influenza both to their allies and to their enemies. That pandemic killed more people than the war itself. Today the state of farming practices and disease surveillance around the world directly influences the prospects for the emergence of a novel strain of influenza with pandemic potential. We are now one world with one health.

We've come to understand more about the development and progression of influenza pandemics than could have been imagined in 1918. The technical capacity exists to rapidly identify and characterize new strains of virus, share scientific information, and produce vaccines and antiviral medications. We understand how a pandemic spreads and how its pace may be controlled or limited.

What will this knowledge give us? In science, industry, and medicine, we have a love affair with knowledge, but this relationship delivers mixed benefits. We love cars but haven't come to terms with global warming. We've had a century of success using antibiotics to treat human infectious disease. Yet, we constantly struggle with antibiotic resistance, and many contend that the past few decades have seen these drugs often used inappropriately.

Sometimes humanity brandishes its cleverness like a great burning torch only to discover that we've set the house on fire, so we must carefully consider the limitations and fickleness of knowledge. We know what public health and other responses to a pandemic are possible, but we must be mindful of the costs in social disruption and other possible consequences.

The benefits of human knowledge tend to distribute themselves to the wealthiest parts of humanity: it is easier for more affluent countries to devote resources to pandemic planning, animal health measures, disease surveillance, and stockpiling of relevant materials. We, as Canadians, will get some of the first doses of vaccines. The reality of an influenza pandemic, however, is that risky animal farming practices in poor subsistence farms on the other side of the world increase the entire world's risk of experiencing an influenza pandemic. When the initial human clusters of cases of a novel strain of influenza appear, we hope to collectively contain it, wherever in the world that occurs. For rich countries to share the fruits and products of knowledge with poor countries makes a lot of sense, but we don't have a good track record of doing this.

Knowledge can be dangerously confused with prediction. We know the issues and principles surrounding an influenza pandemic. Meanwhile, the deeper our understanding, the more we realize that many details cannot be predicted. Knowledge creates our current high level of global concern for a pandemic and gives us an unprecedented chance for preparation. The media message is that a pandemic is on our doorstep. Although it may be correct to say that it is at the door, we don't know when it will decide to knock. It may sit on the stoop for a while. One problem when knowledge becomes confused with prediction is that the failure of prediction may lead people to think that the knowledge is faulty.

The human race is greatly enthusiastic about what knowledge can do; it is less excited when it comes to what knowledge tells us we can't do. This is our collective blind spot when it comes to our love affair with science. When the next influenza pandemic arrives, the impact may be large and far-reaching, and we won't be able to make it go away or prevent every single death. To a large degree, it will run its course; doctors, nurses, public health workers, and society will do their best to mitigate its effects, and their work has the best chance of being appropriate and effective if we understand that some things can be done and some can't. Our understanding of influenza pandemics needs to include a realization that many issues are beyond our control, and a clear eye for these elements is just as important as an appreciation of what actions we can appropriately take.

We live in an era in which an unprecedented richness of science and knowledge results in society setting its expectations at the highest point. Especially in affluent countries, the consideration of a threat to human health is accompanied by the opinion that some doctor or scientist should know how to "do something," in order to "deal with it." However, the next pandemic will not be a purely medical or scientific phenomenon. It will play itself out in societies of human beings, with all our faults and foibles. The challenge is often not whether knowledge exists, but whether the human decisions to understand and use knowledge correspond well with the opportunities for meaningful action.

No matter what, the large majority of people in the world will survive the next influenza pandemic, and human civilization will continue upon its course following this event. Plans surrounding the threat of pandemic influenza are aimed at mitigating the human and societal costs of a pandemic, slowing its progression, and possibly even delaying or averting it. The question of how best to use our knowledge to prepare for and respond to pandemic influenza is a challenge of human judgment, honest communication, and commitment to delivering fair benefits to as many people as possible.

Hopefully, it will be some time before we must address the consequences of the next influenza pandemic, but the timing may not be ours to dictate. We should strive toward being able to say at any point, if a pandemic begins, that we have done what is possible and reasonable to understand its threat, to delay its occurrence, and minimize its impact upon humanity.

GLOBAL HEALTH ORGANIZATIONS

World Health Organization (WHO) site on influenza:
http://www.who.int/csr/disease/influenza/en/

World Health Organization (WHO) site on avian influenza:
http://www.who.int/csr/disease/avian_influenza/en/

European Influenza Surveillance Scheme:
http://www.eiss.org/index.cgi

Food and Agriculture Organization of the United Nations:
http://www.fao.org/ag/againfo/subjects/en/health/
diseases-cards/special_avian.html

CANADA: NATIONAL

Public Health Agency of Canada (PHAC) site on current
seasonal influenza statistics and trends:
http://www.phac-aspc.gc.ca/fluwatch/

Public Health Agency of Canada (PHAC) site on pandemic
influenza:
http://www.phac-aspc.gc.ca/influenza/pandemic_e.html

Public Health Agency of Canada (PHAC) site on
avian influenza:
http://www.phac-aspc.gc.ca/influenza/avian_e.html

Canadian Pandemic Influenza Plan:
http://www.phac-aspc.gc.ca/cpip-pclcpi/

Canadian Food Inspection Agency site on avian influenza:
http://www.inspection.gc.ca/english/anima/heasan/disemala/
avflu/avflue.shtml

Health Canada "It's Your Health" website on avian influenza:
http://www.hc-sc.gc.ca/iyh-vsv/diseases-maladies/
avian-aviare_e.html

Government of Canada Influenza Portal:
http://www.influenza.gc.ca/index_e.html

Canadian Paediatric Society: Caring for Kids–general health information for parents on taking care of your sick child:
http://www.caringforkids.cps.ca/whensick/index.htm

CANADA: PROVINCIAL

ALBERTA
http://www.safecanada.ca/province_e.asp?OP=link&topic=193&PID=13

BRITISH COLUMBIA
http://www.safecanada.ca/province_e.asp?OP=link&topic=193&PID=3

MANITOBA
http://www.gov.mb.ca/health/publichealth/cmoh/pandemic.html

NEWFOUNDLAND AND LABRADOR
http://www.safecanada.ca/province_e.asp?OP=link&topic=193&PID=12

NEW BRUNSWICK
http://www.safecanada.ca/province_e.asp?OP=link&topic=193&PID=6

NORTHWEST TERRITORIES
http://www.safecanada.ca/province_e.asp?OP=link&topic=193&PID=7

NOVA SCOTIA
http://www.gov.ns.ca/govt/pandemic/

NUNAVUT
http://www.safecanada.ca/province_e.asp?OP=link&topic=193&PID=8

ONTARIO
http://www.safecanada.ca/province_e.asp?OP=link&topic=193&PID=1

QUEBEC
http://www.msss.gouv.qc.ca/sujets/santepub/pandemie/index.php
?pandemic

PRINCE EDWARD ISLAND
http://www.safecanada.ca/province_e.asp?OP=link&topic=193
&PID=9

SASKATCHEWAN
http://www.safecanada.ca/province_e.asp?OP=link&topic=193
&PID=10

YUKON
http://www.safecanada.ca/province_e.asp?OP=link&topic=193
&PID=11

UNITED STATES

Centers for Disease Control and Prevention (CDC) site on
pandemic influenza:
http://www.cdc.gov/flu/pandemic

Centers for Disease Control and Prevention (CDC) site on
avian influenza:
http://www.cdc.gov/flu/avian

U.S. Department of Health and Human Services site on
pandemic and avian influenza:
http://pandemicflu.gov/

U.S. National Strategy for Pandemic Influenza:
http://www.whitehouse.gov/homeland/pandemic-influenza.html

Center for Disease Research and Policy, University of
Minnesota: http://www.cidrap.umn.edu/

OTHER COUNTRIES OF NOTE

AUSTRALIA
http://www.health.gov.au/internet/wcms/publishing.nsf/Content
/phd-pandemic-plan.htm

UNITED KINGDOM
http://www.dh.gov.uk/PolicyAndGuidance/EmergencyPlanning
/PandemicFlu/fs/en

REFERENCES

CHAPTER 1—INTRODUCTION
1. World Health Organization. SARS Summary Report. http://www.who.int/csr/sars/country/en/ country2003_08_15.pdf
2. World Health Organization. SARS Probable Cases. http://www.who.int/csr/sars/country/table2004_04_21/ en/index.html

CHAPTER 2—THE INFLUENZA PANDEMIC:
WHAT IT IS, WHY IT MATTERS
1. Knobler, S.L., Mack, A., Mahmoud A., Lemon S.M., eds. "The Threat of Pandemic Influenza: Are We Ready?" Workshop Summary, prepared for the Forum on Microbial Threats, Board on Global Health. National Academy of Sciences, 2005.
2. Luke, C.J., Subbarao K. "Vaccines for Pandemic Influenza." *Emerging Infectious Diseases*, 2006. http://www.cdc.gov/ ncidod/EID/v0112n001/ 05–1147.htm.
3. World Health Organization. http://www.who.int/csr/ disease/avian_influenza/country/en/.
4. World Health Organization. http://www.who.int/csr/ disease/influenza/pandemic/en/.
5. Presentation from Dr Mike Purdue, World Health Organization. "Global Challenges To Accurate Surveillance For Zoonotic Viruses: The Highly Pathogenic Avian Influenza Experiences" at the 2006 International Symposium on Emerging Zoonoses in Atlanta
6. Public Health Agency of Canada, Canadian Pandemic Influenza Plan. http://www.phac-aspc.gc.ca/cpip-pclcpi/.

CHAPTER 3—SEASONAL, AVIAN, AND
PANDEMIC INFLUENZA—THE KEY LINKS
1. Public Health Agency of Canada. Canadian Pandemic Influenza Plan. http://www.phacaspc.gc.ca/cpip-pclcpi/.
2. World Health Organization. "WHO Influenza Pandemic Handbook for Journalists," December 2005. http://www.who.int/csr/don/Handbook_influenza_ pandemic_dec05.pdf.

3. Sibbald, B. "Estimates of Flu-related Deaths Rise with New Statistical Models." *Canadian Medical Association Journal* 168 (2003): 761.

4. Thompson, W.W., Shay, D.K., Weintraub, E, *et al.* "Mortality associated with influenza and respiratory syncytial virus in the United States. *Journal of the American Medical Association* 289 (2003): 179–186.

5. US Department of Health and Human Services. Appendix B: Pandemic Influenza Background. USHS Pandemic Influenza Plan, November 2005. http://www.hhs.gov/pandemicflu/plan/.

6. Centre for Diseases Control and Prevention. Efficacy and Effectiveness of Inactivated Influenza Vaccine. http://www.cdc.gov/flu/professionals/vaccination/efficacy.htm.

7. Knobler, S.L., Mack, A., Mahmoud, A., Lemon, S.M., eds. "The Threat of Pandemic Influenza: Are We Ready?" Workshop Summary, prepared for the Forum on Microbial Threats, Board on Global Health. National Academy of Sciences, 2005.

8. Belshe, R.B. "The Origins of Pandemic Influenza: Lessons from the 1918 Virus," *New England Journal of Medicine* 353 (2005): 2209–2211

9. Stöhr, K. and Esveld, M. "Will Vaccines be Available for the Next Influenza Pandemic?" *Science* 306 (5705) (2004): 2195–2196

10. Barry, J.M. *The Great Influenza: The Epic Story of the Deadliest Plague in History*. New York: Penguin, 2004.

CHAPTER 4—WILL HISTORY REPEAT ITSELF?—INFLUENZA PANDEMICS OVER THE CENTURIES

1. Patterson, K.D. *Pandemic influenza 1700–1900: A Study in Historical Epidemiology*. New Jersey: Rowman & Littlefield, 1987.

2. Barry, J.M. *The Great Influenza: The Epic Story of the Deadliest Plague in History*. New York: Penguin, 2004.

3. Barry, J. "The Site of Origin of the 1918 Influenza Pandemic and its Public Health Implications." *Journal of Translational Medicine*. 2(1) (2004): 3.

4. Knobler, S.L., Mack A., Mahmoud A., Lemon S.M., eds. "The Threat of Pandemic Influenza: Are We Ready?" Workshop Summary, prepared for the Forum on Microbial Threats, Board on Global Health. National Academy of Sciences, 2005.

5   Luke, C.J., Subbarao K. "Vaccines for Pandemic Influenza."
    Emerging Infectious Diseases, 2006. http://www.cdc.gov/nci-
    dod/EID/v0112n001/05-1147.htm.

6. Gaydos, J.C., Top F.H., Hodder R.A., Russell P.K. "Swine
    Influenza A Outbreak, Fort Dix, New Jersey, 1976."
    Emerging Infectious Diseases. 2006. http://www.cdc.gov/nci-
    dod/EID/v0112n001/05-0965.htm.

7. Laitin, E.A. and Pelletier, E.M. "The Influenza A/New
    Jersey (Swine Flu) Vaccine and Guillain-Barré Syndrome:
    The Arguments for a Causal Association." (1997)
    www.hsph.harvard.edu/Organizations/DDIL/swineflu.html.

8. Krause, R. "The Swine Flu Episode and the Fog of
    Epidemics." *Emerging Infectious Diseases*, 2006.
    http://www.cdc.gov/ncidod/EID/v0112n001/05-1132.htm.

9. Seneviratne, U. "Guillain-Barré Syndrome," *Postgrad Medical
    Journal*, 76(902) (2000): 774–82.
    http://pmj.bmjjournals.com/cgi/content/full/76/902/774.

10. Ministry of Health and Long-Term Care, Ontario.
    http://www.health.gov.on.ca/english/
    public/program/emu/avian/history.html

11. World Health Organization. "Avian Influenza: Assessing the
    Pandemic Threat." http://www.who.int/csr/disease/
    influenza/en/H5N1-pass.pdf

12. World Health Organization. Summary of SARS Cases.
    http://www.who.int/csr/sars/
    country/table2004_04_21/en/index.html

13. Peiris, J.S., Chu C.M., Cheng V.C., *et al.* "Clinical
    Progression and Viral Load in a Community Outbreak of
    Coronavirus-associated SARS Pneumonia: A Prospective
    Study." *Lancet* 361 (2003): 1767–72.

CHAPTER 5—PHASES OF A PANDEMIC—HOW
A PANDEMIC COMES TO BE

1. Buxton Bridges, C., Katz J.M., Seto W.H., *et al.* "Risk of
    Influenza A (H5N1) Infection Among Health Care Workers
    Exposed to Patients with Influenza A (H5N1)," *Journal of
    Infectious Diseases* 181 (2000): 344–348.

2. Hien, T.T., Liem N.T., Dung N.T., *et al.* "Avian Influenza A
    (H5N1) in 10 patients in Vietnam." *New England Journal of
    Medicine* 350 (2004): 1179–1188.

3. Ungchusak, K., Auewarakul P., Dowell S.F., *et al.* "Probable
    Person-to-Person Transmission of Avian Influenza (H5N1)."
    New England Journal of Medicine 352 (2005): 333–340.

4. Ferguson, N.M., Cummings D.A., Cauchemez S., Fraser C.,

Riley S., Meeyai A., *et al.* "Strategies for Containing an Emerging Influenza Pandemic in Southeast Asia." *Nature* 437 (2005): 209–14.

5. World Health Organization Writing Group. "Nonpharmaceutical Interventions for Pandemic Influenza, National and Community Measures." *Emerging Infectious Disease Journal* 12 (1) (2006). http://www.cdc.gov/ncidod/EID/v0112n00 1/05–1371.htm.

6. Australian Management Plan for Pandemic Influenza, June 2005 version. http://www.health.gov.au/internet/wcms/ Publishing.nsf/Content/phd-pandemic-plan.htm

CHAPTER 6–CONTAINING THE VIRUS

1. St John, R.K., King, A., de Jong, D., *et al.* "Border Screening for SARS." *Emerging Infectious Diseases* 11 (2005): 6–10.

2. World Health Organization Writing Group. "Nonpharmaceutical Interventions for Pandemic Influenza, International Measures." Emerging Infectious Diseases, 2006. http://www.cdc.gov/ncidod/EID/v0112n001/05–1370.htm.

3. Bell, D.M. World Health Organization Working Group on Prevention of International and Community Transmission of SARS. Public health interventions and SARS spread, 2003. *Emerging Infectious Diseases* 10(2004): 1900–6.

4. Mangili, A. and Gendreau, M.A. "Transmission of Infectious Diseases during Commercial Air Travel." *Lancet* 365 (2005): 989–96.

5. Moser M.R., Bender T.R., Margolis, H.S., *et al.* "An Outbreak of Influenza Aboard a Commercial Airliner." *American Journal of Epidemiology* 110 (1979): 1–6.

6. Marsden, A.G. "Influenza Outbreak Related to Air Travel." *Medical Journal of Australia* 179 (2003): 172–3.

7. Olsen, S.J., Chang, H.L., Cheung, T.Y. *et al.* "Transmission of the Severe Acute Respiratory Syndrome on Aircraft." *New England Journal of Medicine* 349 (2003): 2416–2422.

8. Australian Management Plan for Pandemic Influenza, June 2005. http://www.health.gov.au/internet/wcms/ Publishing.nsf/Content/phd-pandemic-plan.htm.

9. UK Department of Health/HPIH&SD/Immunisation Policy, Monitoring & Surveillance UK Health Departments' Influenza Pandemic Contingency Plan, (October 2005 edition). http://www.dh.gov.uk/PolicyAndGuidance/ EmergencyPlanning/PandemicFlu/fs/en

10. Hayden, F., Belshe, R., Villanueva, R., *et al.* "Management of Influenza in Households: A Prospective, Randomized

Comparison of Oseltamivir Treatment with or without Postexposure Prophylaxis." *The Journal of Infectious Diseases* 189 (2004): 440–449.

11. Peters, P.H. Jr, Gravenstein, S., Norwoo,d P., *et al.* "Long-term Use of Oseltamivir for the Prophylaxis of Influenza in a Vaccinated Frail Older Population." *Journal of the American Geriatric Society* 49 (2001): 1025–31.

12. Welliver, R., Monto, A.S., Carewicz, O., *et al.* "Effectiveness of Oseltamivir in Preventing Influenza in Household Contacts: A Randomized Controlled Trial." *Journal of the American Medical Association 285* (2001):748–54.

13. Monto, A.S., Robinson, D.P., Herlocher M.L. *et al.* "Zanamivir in the Prevention of Influenza Among Healthy Adults: A Randomized Controlled Trial." *Journal of the American Medical Association* 282 (1999): 31–5.

14. Hayden, F.G., Atmar, R.L., Schilling, M., *et al.* "Use of the Selective Oral Neuraminidase Inhibitor Oseltamivir to Prevent Influenza." *New England Journal of Medicine* 341 (1999): 1336–43.

15. Monto, A.S., Pichichero M.E., Blanckenberg, *et al.* "Effectiveness of Neuraminidase Inhibitors in Treatment and Prevention of Influenza A and B: Systematic Review and Meta-analyses of Randomized Controlled Trials." *British Medical Journal* 326 (2003): 1235.

16. Moscona, A. "Neuraminidase Inhibitors for Influenza." *New England Journal of Medicine* 353 (2005): 1363–73.

17. Quarantine Act (Canada) available at http://canadagazette.gc.ca/partII/2004/20040324/hml/sor31-e.html and http://lois.justice.gc.ca/en/Q-1/99147.html

18. US Department of Health and Human Services. Appendix E: Legal Authorities. USHS Pandemic Influenza Plan, November 2005. http://www.hhs.gov/pandemicflu/plan/

CHAPTER 7—MAKING PREPARATIONS FOR
SURVIVING A PANDEMIC

1. Knobler, S.L., Mack, A., Mahmoud, A., Lemon, S.M., eds. "The Threat of Pandemic Influenza: Are We Ready?: Workshop Summary, prepared for the Forum on Microbial Threats, Board on Global Health. National Academy of Sciences, 2005.

2. Dr Michael Osterholm, Center for Infectious Disease Research and Policy. http://www.cidrap.umn.edu/cidrap/content/influenza/avian flu/news/aug082005vaccine.html.

3. World Health Organization (WHO). http://www.who.int/ mediacentre/news/releases/2005/pr11/en/.

4. Canadian Immunization Guide 6th edition 2002. http://www.phac-aspc.gc.ca/publicat/cig-gci/index.html.

5. Emergency Management Unit, Ontario Ministry of Health and Long Term Care. http://www.health.gov.on.ca/english/providers/program/emu/emerg_prep/emerg/broc_plan_010606.pdf.

6. World Health Organization (WHO). http://www.who.int/ water_sanitation_health/diseases/diarrhoea/en/.

7. The Honourable Dennis R O'Connor. Report of the Walkerton Inquiry. Ontario Ministry of the Attorney General, 2002. http:// www.attorneygeneral.jus.gov.on.ca/english/about/pubs/walkerton/.

8. MacKenzie, W.R., Hoxie, N.J., Proctor, M.E., *et al.*"A Massive Outbreak in Milwaukee of Cryptosporidium Infection transmitted Through the Public Water Supply." *New England Journal of Medicine* 331 (1994): 161–167. http://content.nejm.org/cgi/content/full/331/3/161.

9. Center for Infectious Disease Research and Policy. http://www.cidrap.umn.edu/cidrap/content/influenza/general/news/dec1305warnings.htm.

CHAPTER 8—THINGS TO DO IN EVERYDAY LIFE TO LIMIT THE SPREAD OF INFLUENZA

1. CBC's *Quirks and Quarks* broadcast on February 25, 1976. http://archives.cbc.ca/ IDCC-1–75–1965–12739/science_technology/influenza/

2. Nelson, J.D. Jails, "Microbes and the Three-foot Barrier." *New England Journal of Medicine* 335 (1996): 885–86.

3. Feigin, R.D., Baker, C., Herwaldt, L.A. *et al.* "Epidemic Meningococcal Disease in an Elementary-school Classroom." *New England Journal of Medicine* 307 (1982): 1255–57.

4. Bean, B., Moore, B.M., Sterner, B., *et al.* "Survival of Influenza Viruses on Environmental Surfaces." *Journal of Infectious Diseases* 146 (1) (1982):47–51.

5. Centers for Disease Control and Prevention. "Guidelines for Hand Hygiene in Health-Care Settings: Recommendations of the Healthcare Infection Control Practices Advisory Committee and the HICPAC/SHEA/APIC/IDSA Hand Hygiene Task Force." *Morbidity and Mortality Weekly Report* 51 (2002) http://www.cdc.gov/mmwr/PDF/rr/rr5116.pdf

6. Centers for Disease Prevention and Control Handwashing Guidelines. http://www.cdc.gov/ncidod/op/handwashing.htm

7. World Alliance for Patient Safety. "WHO guidelines on Hand Hygiene in Health Care (Advanced Draft)." Geneva: World Health Organization, 2005. http://www.who.int/patientsafety/events/05/HH_en.pdf

8. CBC's *Arts National* broadcast on February 6, 1981. http://archives.cbc.ca/IDC-1-75-1965-12709/science_technology/influenza/clip1

9. CBC's "Surviving 'The Spanish Lady'" broadcast April 10th, 2003. http://archives.cbc.ca/IDC-1-75-1965-12705/science_technology/influenza/clip2

CHAPTER 9—CARING FOR OTHERS DURING A PANDEMIC

1. CBC's *The Current* broadcast on June 23, 2005. http://archives.cbc.ca/IDCC-1-75-1965-12721/science_technology/influenza/

2. Barry, J.M. *The Great Influenza: The Epic Story of the Deadliest Plague in History.* New York: Penguin, 2004.

3. CBC's "Surviving 'The Spanish Lady'" broadcast April 10th, 2003. http://archives.cbc.ca/IDC-1-75-1965-12705/science_technology/influenza/clip2

CHAPTER 10—THE IMPORTANCE OF ANIMAL HEALTH TO HUMAN HEALTH

1. Dr David Nabarro on CBC News online, March 9, 2006. http://www.cbc.ca/story/world/national/2006/03/09/bird-flu-americas060309.html

2. Dr Lonnie King, Centers for Disease Control and Prevention (CDC) "The Convergence of Human and Animal Health: The Dilemma of Connectivity" presentation at the 2006 International Symposium on Emerging Zoonoses, Atlanta.

3. Center for Disease Prevention and Control. Update: Multistate Outbreak of Monkeypox—Illinois, Indiana, Kansas, Missouri, Ohio, and Wisconsin, 2003. *Morbidity and Mortality Weekly Report* 52(27)(2003): 642–646. http://www.cdc.gov/mmwr/preview/mmwrhtml/mm5227a5.htm.

4. Dr Leslie Dierauf, Wildlife Veterinarian, National Wildlife Health Center "Migratory Birds: Victim or Vector?" Presentation at the 2006 International Conference on Emerging Infectious Diseases, Atlanta.

5. National Wildlife Health Center, United States Geological Survey, Highly Pathogenic Avian Influenza, Frequently Asked Questions. http://www.nwhc.usgs.gov/ disease_information/avian_influenza/frequently_ asked_questions.jsp#3b.

6. *The New Scientist*, October 26th, 2004. http://www.newscientist.com/article.ns?id=dn6575

7. Jacques Diof, Food and Agriculture Organization of the United Nations. http://www.examiner.com-/Health_Austrian_Cats_Polish_Swans_Have_Bird_Flu.html.

8. Webster R.G., Hulse, D.J. "Microbial Adaptation and Change: Avian Influenza." *Rev. Sci. Tech. Off Int. Epiz* 23 (2004): 453–65.

9. Food and Agriculture Organization of the United Nations. http://www.fao.org/ag/againfo /subjects/en/health/ diseases-cards/avian_cats.html.

CHAPTER II—THE RACE FOR A PANDEMIC VACCINE

1. CBC's "The Asian Flu arrives in Canada" broadcast on September 19th, 1957. http://archives.cbc.ca/400d.asp?id= 1-75-1965-12707.

2. Public Health Agency of Canada. Frequently Asked Questions on Vaccine Safety. http://www.phac-aspc.gc.ca/ im/vs-sv/vs-faq_e.html.

3. 2005 Oxford County, Ontario Rubella Outbreak. http://new.county.oxford.on.ca/site/1068/default.aspx.

4. United Nations UNICEF on measles deaths yearly. http://www.unicef.org/immunization/index_control.html.

5. Neirynck, S., Deroo, T., Saelens, X., *et al.* "A Universal Influenza A Vaccine Based on the Extracellular Domain of the M2 Protein." *Nature Medicine* 5(10)(1999): 1157–63.

6. Kilbourne, E.D., Couch, R.B., Kasel, J.A., *et al.* "Purified Influenza A Virus N2 Neuraminidase Vaccine is Immunogenic and Non-Toxic in Humans." *Vaccine* 13 (1995):1799–803.

7. Li, Z.N., Mueller, S.N., Ye, L., *et al.* "Chimeric Influenza Virus Hemagglutinin Proteins Containing Large Domains of the Bacillus Anthracis Protective Antigen: Protein Characterization, Incorporation into Infectious Influenza Viruses, and Antigenicity." *Journal of Virology* 79 (2005): 10003–12.

8. US Food and Drug Administration (FDA) Investigational New Drug (IND). www.fda.gov/cder/regulatory/ applications/ind_page_1.htm

9. U.S. Food and Drug Administration (FDA) Emergency Use Authorization of Medical.

http://www.fda.gov/cber/gdlns/emeruse.pdf

10. Palese, P. "Making Better Influenza Virus Vaccines?" *Emerging Infectious Diseases*, 2006. http://www.cdc.gov/ncidod/EID/v0112n001/05-1043.htm

11. Dr Michael Osterholm, Center for Infectious Disease Research and Policy. http://www.cidrap.umn.edu/cidrap/content/influenza/avianflu/news/aug082005vaccine.html

12. Public Health Agency of Canada. Annex D: Recommendations for Pandemic Vaccine Use in a Limited Supply Situation from the Canadian Pandemic Influenza Plan. www.phac-aspc.gc.ca/cpip-pclcpi

13. US Department of Health and Human Services. Appendix D: NVAC/ACIP Recommendations for Prioritization of Pandemic Influenza Vaccine and NVAC Recommendations on Pandemic Antiviral Drug Use. USHS Pandemic Influenza Plan, November 2005. http://www.hhs.gov/pandemicflu/plan/

14. CBC's "The Swine Flu Fiasco" broadcast on February 21st, 1983. http://archives.cbc.ca/IDC-1-75-1965-12711/science_technology/influenza/clip5

CHAPTER 12—THE TRUTH ABOUT
ANTIVIRAL MEDICATIONS

1. Centers for Disease Control and Prevention 2006. CDC Recommends against the Use of Amantadine and Rimantadine for the Treatment or Prophylaxis of Influenza in the United States during the 2005–06 Influenza Season. http://www.cdc.gov/flu/han011406.htm.

2. Jefferson, T., Demicheli V., Rivetti D., *et al.* "Antivirals for Influenza in Healthy Adults: Systematic Review." *Lancet* 367 (2006): 303–13.

3. Moscona, A. "Neuraminidase Inhibitors for Influenza." *New England Journal of Medicine* 353 (2005): 1363–73.

4. Kaiser, L., Wat, C., Mills, T., *et al.* "Impact of Oseltamivir Treatment on Influenza-related Lower Respiratory Tract Complications and Hospitalizations." *Archives of Internal Medicine* 163 (2003): 1667–1672.

5. Commonwealth Scientific and Industrial Research Organization. CSIRO based drug effective against bird flu. http://www.csiro.au/files/mediaRelease/mr2004/PrBirdFlu5.htm

6. Roche. www.roche.com/med-div-2006-01-20.htm

7. Trampuz, A., Prabhu, R.M., Smith, T.F., Baddour, L.M. "Avian Influenza: A New Pandemic Threat?" *Mayo Clinic*

Proceedings 79 (2004): 523–530. [Erratum, Mayo Clin Proc 79 (2004): 833.]

8. Cooper, N.J., Sutton, A.J., Abrams, K.R., *et al.* "Effectiveness of Neuraminidase Inhibitors in Treatment and Prevention of Influenza A and B. Systematic Review and Meta-Analyses of Randomised Controlled Trials." *British Medical Journal* 326 (2003): 1235–1235

9. Hayden, F.G., Gubareva, L.V., Monto, A.S., *et al.* "Inhaled Zanamivir for the Prevention of Influenza in Families." *New England Journal of Medicine* 343 (2000): 1282–1289.

10. Hayden, F.G., Belshe, R., Villanueva, C., *et al.* "Management of Influenza in Households: A Prospective, Randomized Comparison of Oseltamivir Treatment With or Without Postexposure Prophylaxis." *Journal of Infectious Diseases* 189 (2004): 440–449.

11. Welliver, R., Monto, A.S., Carewicz, O., *et al.* "Effectiveness of Oseltamivir in Preventing Influenza in Household Contacts: A Randomized Controlled Trial." *Journal of the American Medical Association* 285 (2001):748–754.

12. Monto, A.S., Robinson, D.P., Herlocher, M.L., Hinson, J.M. Jr, Elliott, M.J., Crisp, A. "Zanamivir in the Prevention of Influenza Among Healthy Adults: A Randomized Controlled Trial." *Journal of the American Medical Association* 282 (1999): 31–35

13. Hayden, F.G., Atmar, R.L., Schilling, M., *et al.* "Use of the Selective Oral Neuraminidase Inhibitor Oseltamivir to Prevent Influenza." *New England Journal of Medicine* 341 (1999): 1336–43.

14. De Jong, Thanh T.T., Khanh T.H., *et al.* "Oseltamivir Resistance during Treatment of Influenza A (H5N1) Infection." *New England Journal of Medicine* 353 (2005): 25–30.

15. *San Francisco Chronicle*. June 24th, 2005. http://www.sfgate.com/cgi-bin/article.cgi?file=/c/a/2005/06/24/mnghtde8lg1.dtl.

16. Forbes.com, November 16th, 2005. http://www.forbes.com/markets/feeds/afx/2005/11/16/afx2339778.html

17. *New York Times*, October 14th, 2005. http://www.nytimes.com/2005/10/14/health/14virus.html?ex=1286942400&en=35e641cfaaceeb9b&ei=5090&partner=rssuserland&emc=rss.

18. Public Health Agency of Canada. Canadian Pandemic Plan. Annex E: Planning Recommendations for the Use of

Antivirals (Anti-Influenza Drugs) in Canada During a
Pandemic. www.phacaspc.gc.ca/cpip-pclcpi.

19. *The Weekend Australian*, March 1ˢᵗ, 2006. http://www.theaus-
tralian.news.com.au/common/story_page/
0,5744,18311882%255E23289,00.html.

CHAPTER 13—IT'S NOT SO SIMPLE: ETHICAL
DILEMMAS DURING AN INFLUENZA PANDEMIC

1. Greenberg, L., *The National Post*. February 21st, 2006.
   "Pandemic Ontario's Emergency Powers Worry MDs: May
   Be Forced Into Work."

2. Health Protection and Promotion Act R.S.O. 1990, Chapter
   H.7, Ontario. http://www.e-Laws.gov.on.ca/DBLaws/
   Statutes/English/90h07_e.htm.

3. Quarantine Act, Canada. http://laws.justice.gc.ca/en/
   Q-1/index.html.

4. Svoboda T., Henry B., Shulman L., *et al.* "Public Health
   Measures to Control the Spread of Severe Acute Respiratory
   Syndrome During the Outbreak in Toronto." *New England
   Journal of Medicine* 350 (2004): 2352–61.

5. University of Toronto Joint Centre for Bioethics Pandemic
   Influenza Working Group. Stand on Guard for Thee:
   Ethical considerations in Preparedness Planning for
   Pandemic Influenza, November 2005.

6. Bill 56: An Act to amend the Emergency Management Act,
   the Employment Standards Act, 2000 and the Workplace
   Safety and Insurance Act, 1997. Ontario Legislative
   Assembly. http://www.ontla.on.ca/documents/Bills/
   38_Parliament/session2/b056_e.htm.

7. Upshur, R., from "Doctors Decry Changes to Emergencies
   Act." http://www.news.utoronto.ca/inthenews/
   archive/2006_02_22.html.

8. Moscona, A. "Neuraminidase Inhibitors for Influenza." *New
   England Journal of Medicine* 353 (2005): 1363–1373.

9. Canadian International Development Agency news release,
   April 23rd, 2004. Canadian Malaria Initiative to Save the
   Lives of Thousands of African Children.
   http://www.acdi-cida.gc.ca/cida_ind.nsf/vall/
   ac98ce0db7e195a985256e7f004980e4?OpenDocument.

10. Knobler, S., Mahmoud, A., Lemon, S., *et al.* eds, Forum on
    Microbial Threat. *Learning from SARS: Preparing for the Next
    Disease Outbreak—Workshop Summary*. Washington: National
    Academies Press, 2004.

11. The Conference Board on Canada. The Economic Impact

of SARS. http://www.dfait-maeci.gc.ca/mexico-city/
economic/may/sarsbriefMay03.pdf.

CHAPTER 14—PRACTICAL PROBLEMS OF AN
INFLUENZA PANDEMIC
1. Barry, J.M. *The Great Influenza: The Epic Story of the Deadliest Plague in History.* New York: Penguin, 2004.
2. McKibbin, W.J., Sidorenko, A.A. "Global Macroeconomic Consequences of a Pandemic Influenza," Lowy Institute for International Policy, February 2006.

PERMISSIONS

The quotations on page 94 are from the CBC television news originally broadcast on April 10, 2003. Courtesy of the Canadian Broadcasting Corporation

The quotation on page 154 is from the CBC radio program *Quirks and Quarks* originally broadcast on February 25, 1976. Courtesy of the Canadian Broadcasting Corporation

The quotation on page 181 is from the CBC radio program *The Current* originally broadcast on June 23, 2005. Courtesy of the Canadian Broadcasting Corporation

The quotation on page 233 is from the CBC television news originally broadcast on September, 29, 1957. Courtesy of the Canadian Broadcasting Corporation

We wish to thank our families and friends for their support during what has been a fast-paced, exciting, and demanding project. Dr. Lam would like especially to express his gratitude to his wife, Margarita, and his son, Theodore, for putting up with the large proportion of his waking hours being spent at his keyboard while working on this book with Dr. Lee. Rosalie Lam and Catherine Antoniades provided invaluable care of Theodore, without which this book could not have been completed on time. Dr. Lee would like to thank his parents, Peter Lee and Teresa Au-Yong for encouraging and supporting him in this endeavour. The authors are grateful to Andrew Lam for his background research. We are appreciative of the early review and feedback upon this book by Margaret Atwood, Graeme Gibson, Dr. Charles Gardner, Richard Munter, and Marco Antoniades. Thanks especially to Margaret Atwood for nudging us along when needed.

We tip our hats to our publisher, Maya Mavjee, for going out on a limb with us, our agent, Anne McDermid, for making sure it all happened, her excellent associate, Martha Magor, and our editor, Amy Black, who pulled it all together.

Both Dr. Lam and Dr. Lee would like to acknowledge the health institutions that we work with and express our appreciation for the lessons that our medical work has taught us. Dr. Lee would like especially to thank his colleagues in Ontario's public health system for their support on this project. We are indebted to our colleagues at the Simcoe Muskoka District Health Unit and at the emergency departments of the Royal Victoria Hospital of Barrie, Ontario, and Toronto East General Hospital. Many of our fellow physicians went out of their way to give us enough flexibility in our schedules to complete this project, and we are grateful to them. All are committed, as we are, to delivering both the best possible health care and the highest quality of health information available to Canadians.

military
influenza outbreaks among, 46–47, 51
spread of other illnesses, 155
monkey pox, 215
Monto, Dr. Arnold S., 69
mucous membranes, 156–57, 173–74, 175

N
N proteins, 30–31
Nabarro, David, 213
nausea, 209
neighbours
caring for those who fall ill, 193–98, 198–206
as support system, 149–50
Netherlands
H7N7 outbreak, 35
vaccination of poultry, 226
New Zealand, travel measures, 104–5
Nigeria, H5N1 outbreak, 34
nurses
infected by SARS, 3, 4–5
killed by Spanish flu, 46

O
Oliva, Dr. Otavio, 99
1 metre rule. *See* social distancing
Ontario
Bill 56, 278–80
Health Protection and Promotion Act, 272–73
Ontario Family Emergency Plan, 135
oral rehydration solutions, 207–8
oseltamivir (Tamiflu). *See* antiviral drugs

P
pandemic influenza, 12–26
age distribution of deaths, 38, 39–40, 58–59, 242, 283–84
containment and treatment, 17–19. *See also* containment measures
criteria, 36
death rates, 19–20
definition, 12–13
differences from SARS, 66–67
differences from seasonal influenza, 38, 39–40, 183–84
obstacles to producing vaccines, 233–34

prevention and treatment, 62–64, 252–53
relationship to avian and seasonal strains, 39–41
treatment with antiviral drugs, 251, 252–53, 258
virulence changes over time, 39–40, 61–62
See also Asian flu; Hong Kong flu; influenza pandemics; Spanish flu
pandemic phases, 14, 52, 58, 61, 71–92
cyclical nature, 91–92
interpandemic period, 72–73, 84–85, 91
pandemic alert period, 73–80, 84–85
pandemic period, 81–88, 86–87
pandemics, definition, 35–36
Pedialyte, 207
personal habits. *See* cough and sneeze etiquette; handwashing; social distancing
personal preparations, 121–52
annual flu shots, 125–26
cooking poultry thoroughly, 129
emergency supplies, 135–47
end-of-life planning, 148–49
handwashing. *See* handwashing
personal health, 129, 130–35
pneumovax vaccine, 126
travel to affected countries, 128–29
pets, 227–29
Pfeiffer, Richard, 47
pharmaceutical industry, 237–38. *See also* GlaxoSmithKline; Roche
pigs, as "mixing vessel" for viruses, 32–33
pneumonia, 46, 63, 126, 189–90
pneumovax vaccine, 126
polio, 78, 128, 234
The Politics of Fear (Furedi), 24
poultry
commercial farming, 218–19, 221–22, 224, 225–26
contact with humans, 35, 73, 222
cooking thoroughly, 129
culling, 34, 91, 213–14, 221, 223, 288–89
free-range, 217–18, 222
safety of eating, 226–27
vaccination, 224, 225–26

prairie dogs, 215
pregnant women, increased susceptibility to pandemic influenza, 38, 59–60, 146
privacy, right to, 272
public gatherings
    avoiding, 162–63, 166
    restrictions and cancellations, 83, 85, 94, 115
public health agencies
    definition of public health, 69
    ethical dilemmas, 271
    focus on Pandemic Alert Period, 89
    importance of open communication, 64–66, 90, 306, 307, 308
    preparedness, 89–91
    responsibilities, 70–71
Public Health Service Act (U.S.), 117
public transit, 143, 160, 165, 166, 167–68, 176

Q
quarantine, 113–15, 154, 272–74
    difference from isolation, 76, 110
    economic and social costs, 273–74, 294
    legislation, 117–18, 272–73
    in Phase 3, 76
    in Phase 5, 79
    in Phase 6, 81, 82
    of SARS patients, 3–4, 8, 112
    during Spanish flu pandemic, 273–74
    of travellers, 102–5

R
radios, 142
rate and effort of breathing, 201–2, 204–5
rationing, 83, 280–87
    of antiviral drugs, 18–19
    of medical care, 59–60, 280–84
    of medical equipment, 282–83
    of vaccines, 59–60
relative immunity, 197
Relenza. See antiviral drugs
respiratory hygiene. See cough and sneeze etiquette
reverse genetics, 240
Rimantadine. See antiviral drugs
RNA viruses, 29–30
Roche, 255–57, 264, 284

Rome, ancient, 43–44, 48
rubella, 234–35
Russia
    increase in diphtheria cases, 234
    vaccination of poultry, 226
Russian flu, 49

S
safer sex, 133, 134
Sardo, William, 291
SARS, 3–9, 30
    containment of, 3–4, 5–6, 8, 69, 111–12
    differences from influenza, 66–67
    economic disruption, 4, 289
    eradication, 5–6
    global impact, 312–13
    health care workers infected by, 3, 4–5, 275, 297
    impact on health care systems, 3, 4–5, 7–8, 97, 295–300
    inability to prepare for, 8, 9
    mask wearing during Toronto outbreak, 177
    screening of travellers, 102
    social disruption, 3–4, 8
    spread on airplanes, 103
    statistics, 3, 5, 66
    Toronto outbreak, 3–5, 7–8
    travel health alert notices issued, 101
    "work quarantine" strategy, 115
Schabas, Dr. Richard, 260
school closings, 83, 85, 115, 169–71
seasonal influenza, 8, 28–33, 236
    age distribution of deaths, 29, 38, 39–40, 59
    contagiousness, 114
    differences from pandemic influenza, 38, 39–40, 183–84
    monitoring and treatment, 72
    relationship to avian and pandemic strains, 39–41
    spread on airplanes, 103
    statistics, 28
    symptoms compared with common cold, 29
    treatment with antiviral drugs, 250–51, 255, 263–64
    types of viruses, 29–33
    vaccines, 28, 31–32, 125–26, 233, 239

341

self-isolation, 85, 115
"self-shielding," 85, 116, 170
"sentinel physicians," 75
severe acute respiratory syndrome (SARS). *See* SARS
shaking hands, avoiding, 162–63, 164–65
shortness of breath, 189–90, 201–2, 204–5
Silverstein, Dr. Arthur, 245–46
smallpox, 30, 35, 128, 234
smoking, 130–32
smuggling, of exotic animals, 215–17
"snow days," 85, 116, 169–71, 294
social distancing, 154, 155, 164–65, 166–68, 195
    effectiveness compared with mask wearing, 175–76
    within the home, 168–69, 191–92
Spanish flu, 12, 45–47, 49
age distribution of deaths, 59
    combined with bacterial illnesses, 63
    containment measures, 94, 96, 104–5, 106
    death rate, 14, 19, 20, 47, 120–21
    deaths from dehydration, 181–82
    effectiveness of quarantine, 273–74
    genetic sequencing of virus, 37
    global spread, 313
    mask wearing during pandemic, 174, 175
    "mild" wave, 45–46, 58
    mutation of virus, 62
    second wave, 45–46
    social disruption, 88
    third and fourth waves, 47
    unusual symptoms, 184
    virulence, 39
    West Coast less affected than East, 60
sports drinks, 207
Streptococcus pneumoniae, 126
subunit vaccination, 240
swine flu, 44, 49, 51–53, 64, 244–47
    vaccine, 52–53

T
Tamiflu. *See* antiviral drugs
telephone hotlines, 79, 182, 183, 216, 301, 302
telephones, 142

temperature, 198–200, 201, 204–5, 209
tetanus shots, 145, 234
Thailand
    H5N1 spread between humans, 74
    travel measures during SARS outbreak, 101
thermometers, 199–200
Toronto, SARS outbreak, 3–5, 7–8, 273, 275, 289
tourism, 4, 97, 289, 294–95
trade, disruption by a pandemic, 21, 80, 135–36, 293–95
travel measures, 94–109
    border closures, 17, 95–97, 101–2, 106–7, 272, 289, 306–7
    within a country, 106
    peak effectiveness, 95, 97–98
    in Phase 5, 79–80
    in Phase 6, 83, 87
    quarantine of travellers, 102–5
    during SARS outbreak, 8
    screening of travellers, 101–2, 272
    during Spanish flu pandemic, 94, 96, 104–5, 106
    travel advisories, 105–6, 128, 129, 289
    travel health alert notices, 101
travel, to H5N1-affected countries, 128–29
tuberculosis, 155, 272
turmeric extract, 147–48
Turner, Susanna, 291

U
United Kingdom
    army stricken by Spanish flu, 47
    navy stricken by Spanish flu, 46
    pandemic plan, 105–6
United States
    army stricken by Spanish flu, 46
    army stricken by swine flu, 51
    Asian flu outbreak, 50
    availability of flu vaccines, 63
    community-based containment measures, 116
    estimated impact of influenza pandemic, 56–57
    Hong Kong flu outbreak, 51
    pandemic plan, 56–57, 116, 170, 174, 241–43, 259, 294

VINCENT LAM was born in London, Ontario. He trained in medicine at the University of Toronto and works as an emergency physician in Toronto. Dr. Lam is a writer whose recent book of fiction, *Bloodletting and Miraculous Cures*, has been received with critical acclaim and has been dramatized for broadcast by CBC Radio. Dr. Lam's non-fiction writing has appeared in the *University of Toronto Medical Journal*, the *Globe and Mail*, the *National Post*, and *Toronto Life* magazine. Dr. Lam lives in Toronto with his wife, Margarita, and his son, Theodore. He escapes urban life periodically to work as a ship's doctor in the Arctic and the Antarctic and to spend time at the family cottage on Georgian Bay.

COLIN LEE was born in Malaysia. He learned his craft at the University of Toronto, McGill University, and the London School of Hygiene and Tropical Medicine in England. Dr. Lee specializes as a public health physician and an emergency physician north of Toronto, where he concentrates on the control of infectious diseases. He is currently appointed to Ontario's Provincial Infectious Disease Advisory Committee and is actively involved in local and provincial pandemic influenza planning. Dr. Lee's public health expertise and interest in global health and culture have taken him to developing countries in Africa and Asia, where he has collaborated on malaria and HIV/AIDS prevention initiatives. His annual expeditions as a ship's doctor in the Arctic and the Antarctic allow him to enjoy Mother Nature's breathtaking beauty and tranquility.